InfeXBloc™ – Building a Shield for Mom

Senior Care - Regaining trust after the COVID-19 storm

Ashish Warudkar
ashish@InfeXBloc.com

Table of Contents

FOREWORD **6**

CHAPTER 1: HOW DID WE GET HERE AND HOW DO WE NAVIGATE THROUGH THIS STORM? **11**

    LONG-TERM ISSUES EXPOSED 11
    LOCKDOWNS ARE NOT SUSTAINABLE 12
    AREAS OF GREATEST RISK IN THE AGE OF CORONAVIRUS 13
    WHAT ABOUT TESTING? 13
    WHAT ABOUT CONTACT TRACING? 14
    COMMISSIONS OF INQUIRY! 15
    THE EMERGING TRUST DEFICIT 16
    REBUILDING TRUST 16
    GOALS VS STRATEGY VS TACTICS VS TOOLS 17
        A New Way of Thinking 17
        Leveraging distributed architectures 18
        From fragile to anti-fragile 20

CHAPTER 2: LESSONS FROM THE PAST - FROM AIRLINES TO CYBERSECURITY **22**

CHAPTER 3: FOUNDATIONS OF SAFETY – HAZARDS, CONTROLS, SWISS CHEESE, AND RISK **24**

    PREDICTABLE VS UNPREDICTABLE 25
    THE OCCUPATIONAL RISK PYRAMID 27
    THE HIERARCHY OF CONTROLS 29
    THE SWISS CHEESE MODEL 29
    SAFETY AS CAPACITY 31
    HFACS 33

CHAPTER 4: HAZARD IDENTIFICATION **34**

    SENIOR CARE IS A COMPLEX ECOSYSTEM 34
        From outside 35
        When the bug is inside 35
        The aerial pathway 36
        Telemetry of the spread 39
    THIS IS NOT NEW KNOWLEDGE 40
    THE 800-POUND GORILLA IN OUR LIVING ROOM 42
    COMPLEX SYSTEMS ARE GNARLY! 43

CHAPTER 5: OVERCOMING THIS CHALLENGE WITH INFEXBLOC™ **45**

    STATICS -VS- DYNAMICS 45
    CONCEPTUAL UNDERPINNINGS OF INFEXBLOC™ 45
        Introducing friction 45
        Provable and Repeatable process 46
        Implicit Trust policy 46
        Proven Trust policy 47
        A strong community perimeter 47
        Resident room perimeter 48
        Defining 'Proven trust' 49
    IMPLEMENTATION OF INFEXBLOC™ - LEVERAGING TECHNOLOGY 49

- *Using a unified entrance complex* 50
- *Using an access-id card for each entrant* 50
- *Using an 'InfeXPASS™' encrypted access-id* 50
- *Using enforcement of PPE utilization* 51
- *Using automated sliding doors for resident rooms* 51
- *Using equipment to resist aerial transmission* 51
- *Defining an 'InfeXCON™' status for the community* 51
- *Integrated authentication and authorization* 52
- *The community will have 'black boxes'* 53
- *Correlate the resident billing to the community InfeXCON™ status* 53
- IMPLEMENTING CHANGE MANAGEMENT 53
- IMPLEMENTING THE INFEXBLOC SCORECARD™ 54
- IMPLICATIONS OF DEPLOYING INFEXBLOC™ ARCHITECTURE 54
  - *On community owners, operators and investors* 54
  - *On architects & designers* 55
  - *On the process architecture* 55
  - *On the equipment* 56
  - *On the PPE* 56
  - *On caregiver health* 56
  - *On resident's family members* 56
  - *On placement agencies* 57
  - *On residents and the care-service, they receive* 57
  - *On healthcare providers* 57
  - *On non-caregiving staff* 58
  - *On oversight - regulators, inspection (LPA), Ombudsman* 58
  - *On volunteers* 58
  - *On activity staff* 58
  - *On delivery staff* 58
  - *On the cost of care* 58

CHAPTER 6: WHY IS INFEXBLOC™ SAFER? 60

- THE PRISM OF CONTROLS AND SAFEGUARDS 60
- INFEXBLOC™ WORKS AT THREE LEVELS 63
  - *Planning for prevention* 63
  - *Safe Execution* 63
  - *Recovery, when infection enters the community* 64
- QUANTITATIVE ANALYSIS 64
- COMPARATIVE ANALYSIS 67
- CLASSIFYING THE SAFEGUARDS AND CONTROLS OF INFEXBLOC™ 69
- ONE MORE ORBIT AROUND THE EARTH 71
- A LEARNING ORGANIZATION 71

CHAPTER 7 : DELIVERING TRANSPARENCY 72

- MECHANICS OF DELIVERING TRANSPARENCY 74
- SPECIFIC PROPOSALS TO DELIVER TRANSPARENCY 74

CHAPTER 8: CAN WE PROVE THIS? 77

- IS THE THESIS THEORETICALLY SOUND? 77
- HAS THIS THESIS WORKED ELSEWHERE? 77
- CAN WE SIMULATE THIS THESIS? 77
  - *InfeXSIM™ - A new weapon system for the Senior Care Communities* 78
- CAN WE INJECT FAILURE? 79
- CAN WE ESTABLISH THE SOUNDNESS BY DOING PILOT PROJECTS? 79

CHAPTER 9: BENEFITS OF DEPLOYING THE INFEXBLOC™ ARCHITECTURE 80
- For every stakeholder in this industry 80
- For residents and families 80
- For single community operators 80
- For multi-community operators 81
- For DSS & Public health authorities 81
- For Caregivers and Healthcare professionals 81
- For Entrepreneurs, Community Owners, Operators, Investors, and business planners 82
- For Insurance companies 84

CHAPTER 10: CHALLENGES 85

CHAPTER 11: IMPLEMENTATION QUESTIONS 86

CHAPTER 12: DIGITIZATION OF SENIOR CARE 88
- Using real-time dashboards 88
- Publishing a stream of events 92
- Implications for litigation 93
- Implications for Licensing, Oversight, and Human Capital Management 94

CHAPTER 13: FUTURE 95
- Uphill climb ahead 95
- Every industry is reinventing itself 96
- Tomorrow will be better 97
- Applied Theory 97
- Industry Maturity Model 98

CHAPTER 14: A SINCERE HOPE 100

CHAPTER 15: THE CARE OF THE CAREGIVER 101

REFERENCES 102

BIBLIOGRAPHY 105

ABOUT 107

Table of figures

Figure 1 : The world of Senior Care 6
Figure 2 : Gartner's Post Pandemic Planning Framework 8
Figure 3 : InfeXBloc™ is a confluence of many advanced disciplines 9
Figure 4 : The English language is not enough to explain away this disaster! 11
Figure 5 : Coronavirus exploited existing weaknesses 12
Figure 6 : Hospitals became hotspots for Coronavirus infection 14
Figure 7 : Senior care industry was the ground-zero of Coronavirus 16
Figure 8 : Existing Senior care communities shift the infectious cases to hospitals 20
Figure 9 : InfeXBloc™ community will resist the infection spread 20
Figure 10: Nassim Taleb's fragility spectrum 21
Figure 11: Understanding Risk 24
Figure 12: Hienrich's Accident Pyramid 26
Figure 13: Pandemic's Asymmetrical Impact on Seniors 28
Figure 14: Hierarchy of Controls 29
Figure 15: James Reason's Swiss Cheese Model of failure in Complex Systems 30
Figure 16: Safety signage in my childhood town 31
Figure 17: A complex operational ecosystem 34
Figure 18: The complexity multiplies on the inside 36
Figure 19: The aerial route 37
Figure 20: Man sneezing 38
Figure 21: Micro-droplets linger on for a long time 38
Figure 22: Is Coronavirus Airborne? 39
Figure 23: Blacklight simulation of spread telemetry 40
Figure 24: Los Angeles County (source CDSS)[20] 41
Figure 25: GAO Report 42
Figure 26: An example causal loop diagram for the COVID-19 threat 44
Figure 27: Strong perimeter 47
Figure 28: Maximize transmission friction 48
Figure 29: Implementing 'proven trust' 49
Figure 30: Without InfeXBloc™ 61
Figure 31: InfeXBloc™ resists the spread 61
Figure 32: Explained in Safety Engineering terminology 62
Figure 33: Primary, Secondary, Tertiary neighborhoods 62
Figure 34: COVID-19 Restrictions have been very hard on seniors 73
Figure 35: Death from COVID better than from loneliness!! 73
Figure 36: Comparing business model canvas[25] before and after InfeXBloc™ implementation 83
Figure 37: Implementation Framework 86
Figure 38: A real time Safety Dashboard – absence of negatives 88
Figure 39: A real time Safety Dashboard – presence of positives 89
Figure 40: InfeXBloc™ Caregiver Workload Spider Dashboard 90
Figure 41: InfeXBloc™ Resident Journey Map 91
Figure 42: InfeXBloc™ Resident 360 Map 92
Figure 43: Event streams from InfeXBloc™ enabled communities 93
Figure 44: Trust Deficit 95
Figure 45: A 5 level Maturity Model 98

Foreword

In 2020, the business world has changed forever. Massive market forces have been unleashed by the pandemic. Some believe nothing is going to be the same again, others hope the world will go back to normal. We are at an inflection point.

Like an earthquake, a massive amount of energy has been suddenly released. In an earthquake's impact zone, all buildings shake but do so differently depending on their alignment to the seismic waves emerging from the epicenter, their own architecture, and their building materials. Similarly, different businesses have experienced the pandemic differently. Some have actually benefited, but a large number have suffered a devastating impact on their business models.

The world of Senior Care (Figure 1) has changed forever. All 28,000+ Assisted Living communities and 15,000+ Skilled Nursing communities, now have their business model's engine-check light on!

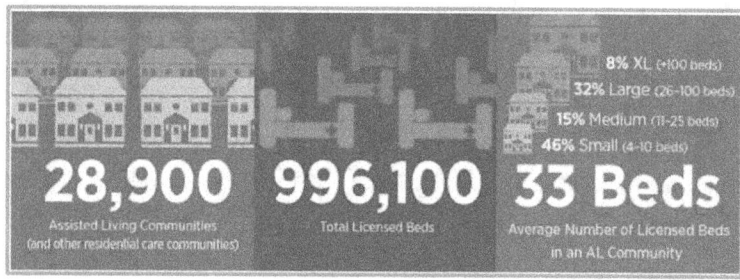

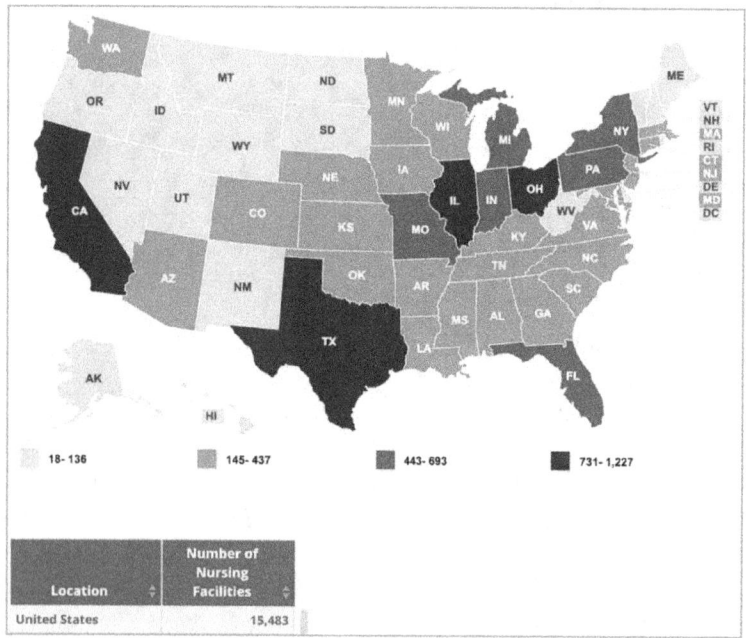

Figure 1 : The world of Senior Care

Your operating costs are hurting your margins, resident and staff departures raise short-term viability questions, your operations contracts could be at risk. The atmosphere of fear is affecting your occupancy, and current residents experience isolation, are upset, and suffer. Your marketing efforts are impaired with many bottlenecks in the pipelines, visitation is restricted, tours - your major differentiator - are shut down. Existing project cashflow assumptions are void, you may have to infuse more capital to save these projects. Future projects are hard to justify, and deal flow has slowed down. The coming tsunami of lawsuits is real – some say that Coronavirus litigation may make its Tobacco and Asbestos predecessors look like child's play. Insurance premiums are escalating 50-60% and not even covering future Coronavirus related claims - future insurability is at risk. Your communities have suffered uncontrolled harm. You are worried!

CDC, State DSS, and the media are not making it any easier, you have lost your autonomy and feel reactive and experience a loss of operational control. Politicians are engaging in their usual bickering. No help is coming for you!

You wish this nightmare was over. You hope the vaccine[30] will do it, but science tells us that there are many factors that determine how long this nightmare could continue[27]. Deep in your gut, you worry that this may not be over anytime soon. You know that the effects on your business model will persist long after the vaccine becomes available. You are nervous and everything you worked hard for is at risk. It's a situation that cannot be ignored or wished away.

How your organization responds to these events, will determine your organization's ability to recover from these events. You can't change history. You must change the future. Yet you are in the present time and trying to understand both what happened and what should happen next. The work of caring for your residents must continue in spite of this catastrophic event. Somehow your organization must figure out a path forward through a very emotional and complicated environment. Decisions must be made. How should you proceed in the face of this uncertainty? What is the right response? What is the right reaction?

Your organization's response must be a deliberate management strategy. There are many victims of this catastrophe. The residents we lost, the present residents, relatives, caregivers, healthcare professionals, management staff, executives, investors. You realize that although you are impacted at a secondary level (Figure 33), but you will be called upon to lead the organization's response to this horrible failure. You will have to determine how tomorrow will look for your organization, how tomorrow will look and how you restore your organization's ability to do high consequence work even better than before the pandemic. You will be called upon to make your organization better[41].

Deep breath time…

You are still the captain, you must lead! You are still required to feel confident that your community will not appear in the negative headlines in the future. You still desire reliable, safe, and stable operations without catastrophic outcomes. A new way of thinking is required. This, is a brand definition opportunity.

In India, where I grew up, a 4.0 earthquake can flatten an entire city and kill thousands, but here in California, I have faced many 7.3+ earthquakes (a thousand times more powerful shaking) without significant damage. Why is this? In India, they build homes with cement and concrete. In the USA, we build with wood. The difference is our anti-fragile approach in the architecture and building materials employed. Our building design absorbs the shocks rather than crumbling because of it.

In order to get better answers, we must ask better questions.
Original question : Who is responsible?

Better question   :   What is responsible?

If we see the Coronavirus problem as an external problem, then we will look for outsiders to provide solutions based on existing thoughts and beliefs. Existing ideas have created this current problem. If we want different results, we must think differently. This book will explore this situation wide and deep. In order for us to restore our ability to do 'high risk high consequence' work better than before the pandemic, a deep assessment is warranted. Instead of looking outside for the cause of our troubles, it will do an 'open-heart-surgery' of our communities. It will put the control stick in our firm hands.

As we strategize on the road ahead for our Senior Care Communities, it is worth pondering over Gartner's "Post Pandemic Planning Framework"[42] (Figure 2). By fall-2020 we are past the 'Respond phase' and must think of the 'Recover' and 'Renew phases'. While different communities may take different pathways in the Recovery and Renewal phases, in this book we offer a strategy that is generally oriented towards the Reinvent and Rescale approaches.

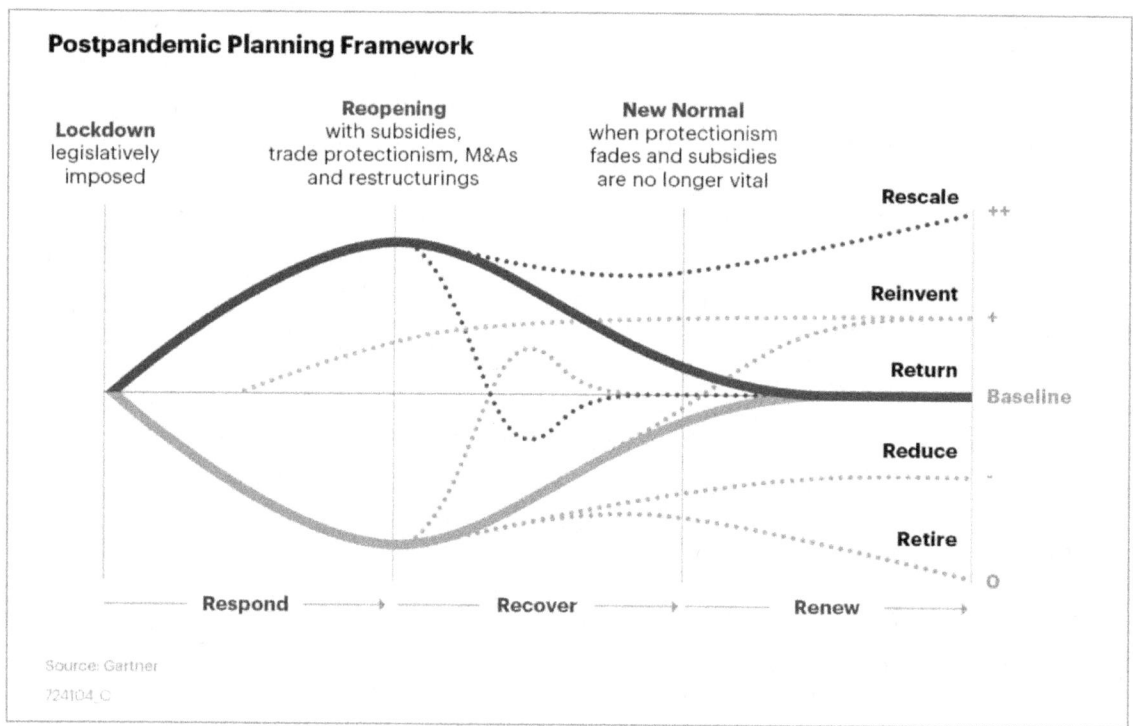

Figure 2 : Gartner's Post Pandemic Planning Framework

What if we could inoculate our business model by making our communities pandemic-resistant and stay attractive to the 2.5 million senior residents today, 4000+ who are turning 85 every day, and the 73 million baby boomers that are coming. If we solve this pandemic problem right, we can get a major bump. If we do nothing, a great opportunity is missed! The choice has shades of "Netflix -v- Blockbuster".

InfeXBloc™ is an operational architecture that was created to solve the problems revealed by the pandemic. While professional building architects typically target the building statics of a community, InfeXBloc™ will combine the static features with the dynamics of operations of a Senior Care community, like the interactions (at run time) between:

- the physical building
- the people operations (staffing, training, caregiving activities, PPE and other safety protocols, kitchen and meals operations, pharmacy fulfillment dynamics, medicine delivery and tracking operations, physician/ nurse/ hospice/ other healthcare visits, relatives and visitors interaction dynamics, prospective resident marketing tours, new resident move-ins, egress to and ingress from hospitals, etc.)

This book takes a multi-disciplinary approach. It is a confluence of ideas from multiple disciplines (Figure 3) including safety and resilience engineering, complex systems thinking, cyber security, cloud native software architectures, digital transformation, building architecture, mechanical engineering and simulation as applied to the problem of resident, caregiver, community and business safety in post-COVID senior care.

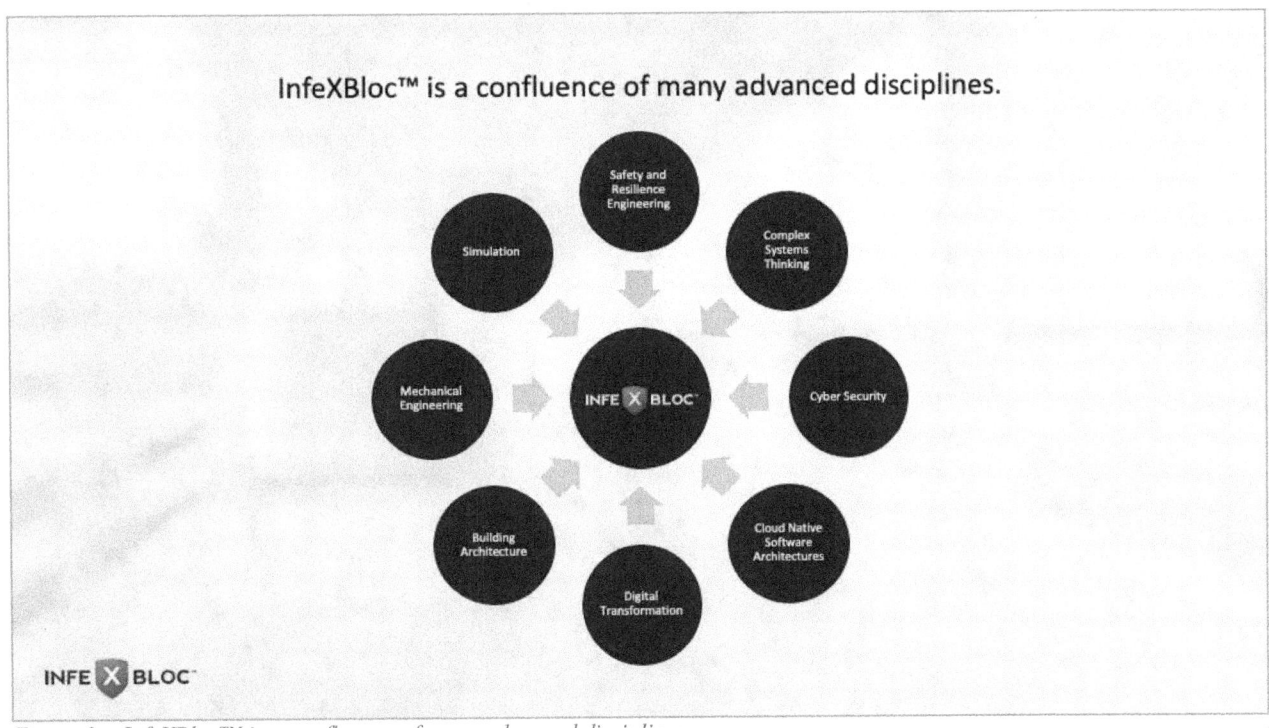

Figure 3 : InfeXBloc™ is a confluence of many advanced disciplines

InfeXBloc™ will not just get us back to a better normal but will also harness these unprecedented market forces and help us thrive by becoming pandemic-resistant. It is an antifragile[16] approach. One of the most critical advantages is that it will allow us to effectively compete with non-consumption[28]. With that nut cracked, we are ready for the silver tsunami.

In the next several years, safety will be the demand driver for our industry.

This book is dedicated to the idea of making our communities pandemic resistant and thus 'Building a Shield for Mom'.

Chapter 1: How did we get here and how do we navigate through this storm?

In California, a senior care community is called an RCFE (Residential Care Faciliities for the Elderly). The focus of these communities is providing a safe environment for seniors, who need a higher level of care than they can receive at home while also relieving the stress from family members. However, by their very nature, these communities also represent target-rich environments for infectious diseases, which can destroy that safety.

While these communities should be defended like nuclear installations, the Coronavirus pandemic has uniquely highlighted the deficiencies in the current model used in this defense. With the severity of the issue now brought to light, there is a new and immediate urgency to examine our practices and improve the outcomes for our residents.

The news headlines of 50,000+ seniors lost (Figure 4) depict a numbing scale of the disaster we have suffered. While the news is focused on sensation (such as the policies that mandated admittance/re-admittance of COVID-19 positive residents to Nursing home communities, shortage of essential PPE supplies and testing gear, choked overseas supply chains, etc.), digging deeper to the root causes of this epic loss of life is far more valuable to ensure our communities and our residents are not put at risk again.

> ♦ WSJ NEWS EXCLUSIVE | U.S.
> ## Coronavirus Deaths in U.S. Nursing, Long-Term-Care Facilities Top 50,000
> A WSJ analysis shows more than 250,000 infection cases among residents and staffers at long-term-care facilities

Figure 4 : The English language is not enough to explain away this disaster!

It's worth noting, that when disaster forensic experts, study catastrophic failure in complex systems, the common thread is multiple fault points in the ecosystem that resulted in a chain of events. This has been borne out in the root cause analysis reports of other epic disasters like the Three-mile Island nuclear accident, the 1986 Challenger disaster, the 9-11 Commission Report, the 2003 Columbia Shuttle disaster, and Hurricane Katrina.

Once again, the truth of that is being borne out – this time in the very communities where we strive to keep our residents safe. In truth, it was not one fault point that led to the loss of life our communities have experienced due to Coronavirus. Instead, multiple fault points combined to result in a system that was both ill-equipped and ill-prepared to combat a highly infectious and deadly disease among the vulnerable population in our communities.

Long-Term Issues Exposed

This book focuses on a deficiency pointed out in the GAO report[1,2] (Figure 5) which found that:

"Most nursing homes and long-term care communities weren't doing enough to protect patients from spreading infection before the coronavirus pandemic. This has been a long-term issue and so the current environment really reinforces the need to focus on these types of infection control measures".

Yet, is it any wonder that the levels of infection control and prevention in communities across our nation was found to be so sadly lacking?

For decades, Federal authorities have delegated the oversight function in our industry to the 50 states. Put simply, this practice produced 50 experiments on a broad spectrum from the strong oversight model (e.g. California) to the relatively lighter oversight found in other states.

Table 2: Infection Prevention and Control Deficiencies Cited, by State, 2017

State	Number of surveyed nursing homes	Number of surveyed nursing homes with an infection prevention and control deficiency cited	Percentage of surveyed nursing homes with an infection prevention and control deficiency cited
AK	16	5	31.3
AL	201	101	50.2
AR	217	86	39.6
AZ	131	30	22.9
CA	1,174	712	60.6
CO	187	87	46.5
CT	213	66	31.0
DC	18	6	33.3

Figure 5 : Coronavirus exploited existing weaknesses

It's important to note, however, that when an industry's self-regulation is found lacking and a catastrophe exposes its vulnerabilities, the pressure on regulators to step in increases. In essence, this makes it is only a matter of time before regulations are introduced, requiring stringent measures to keep our vulnerable residents safe.

Lockdowns Are Not Sustainable

Our first reaction to the Coronavirus pandemic was to go into lockdown. This response was a replica of first reactions in other industries to their emergent events, which eventually were forced to change their practices dramatically to remain viable in a changing world:
- Following September 11, 2001, USA commercial aviation was shut down, a complete lockdown.
- With the advent of public clouds like AWS, Azure, and Google Cloud, enterprise IT departments locked down their data centers, refusing to accept that software application assets could be deployed to public clouds, thus going into lockdown.

It was a pattern that our own industry followed when faced with the new viral threat. Yet, in the matter of only a few months, we have realized that lockdowns in Nursing and Assisted Living Community are simply not sustainable.

The impact of these extended 'shelter-in-place' orders on seniors' psychological health, with escalating feelings of loneliness and despair, even became the focus of a very eye-opening and saddening report[10].

Areas of Greatest Risk in the Age of Coronavirus

Public health experts rank the locations that pose the greatest risk for contracting Coronavirus as follows[15] (ranging from 1 to 10, with 10 being the riskiest):

- Unnamed   10
- Bars and large music concerts   9
- Sports stadiums, gyms, amusement parks, churches, and buffets   8
- Public pools   7
- Movie theaters, hair salons, barbershops   6
- Planes, beaches, bowling alleys and backyard BBQs   5
- Busy city walks and dentist offices   4
- Libraries, museums, grocery stores, hotels, golf courses   3
- Pumping gas, walking/running and biking   2
- Restaurant takeout and tennis   1

Most of the above are typical activities that we as non-residents of Senior Care community engage in on a regular basis (notice rank 10 is unnamed).

However, if we were to rank a list of places our residents are most likely to be exposed to infectious bugs, hospitals would be a 10, and senior care community might be just slightly less risky.

That should not mean though that we simply accept these risks as static, without working to improve the safety we provide. Instead, we must work to dramatically lower the risk ranking for Senior Care community, in order to live up to the promise of care and security that we offer our residents.

What about Testing?

One option that has been proposed to improve safety in our communities is 100% testing. However, the value of this proposal is questionable.

A test result only reflects the status of that resident at that point in time. This means that even if all seniors were tested at any given instant, that metric can become meaningless the next day.

When you add in the consideration that the number of infection propagation vectors (more on this in a later section called 'Senior Care is a complex ecosystem') is astronomical, it becomes clear that one-time testing is not the entire answer.

Even if periodic testing (for example, every week) of all residents is considered, the only value the practice will deliver on its own, is making us aware that one or more of our residents has just tested positive for Coronavirus. So, what could we do with this information?

- Report it to DSS
- From there, we must decide whether or not to move the resident to the hospital. In practical terms, this only results in shifting the location of the infectious resident, a choice that has led to tragic tales from the hospitals in New York[12]. Even during non-pandemic times, hospitals by definition become hotspots for infection, the pandemic exacerbated this problem (Figure 6). By just relocating all COVID-19 positive residents to hospitals, we only further contribute to the hospital overload problem.

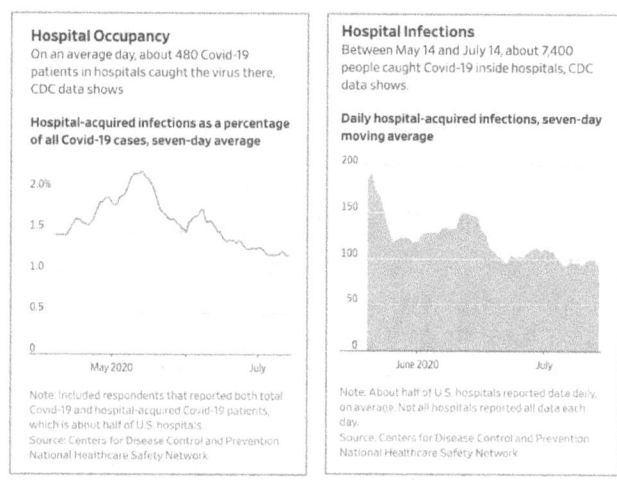

Figure 6 : Hospitals became hotspots for Coronavirus infection

Even worse, none of the above options have done anything to contain the spread and we still have not addressed the underlying infection spread vector in order to ensure the safety of the balance of our seniors.

That's why this book proposes a different solution that will not only inform DSS but also address the need for containment of the virus in our communities and within our communities.

What about contact tracing?

Contact tracing is a forensic tool that attempts to see ahead by looking back. Once a COVID-positive case is detected, contact-tracers try to investigate and plot a graph to determine all the people or places that the patient had been in the last several days and continue these investigative inquiries to multiple levels of depth in the graph. The attempt is to identify the possible 'blast radius' and all those who might be within it.

It is reactive and attempts to execute quarantine procedures on those who might have been in the blast radius. The technique itself is inaccurate at best because it relies on people's memory and willingness to share[29]. It is only effective when the infection has not become widespread, because once that happens, the individual contact graphs intersect and get very diffused. While it may have some effectiveness in the public health domain in the early stages of an epidemic, but its use inside of a senior care community is questionable at best.

Commissions of inquiry!

There is already word of the formation of congressional inquiry commissions to dig into the COVID-19 debacle for seniors. For now, it's fair to conclude that, like in other complex systems, multiple points of failure will be found that resulted in the Coronavirus catastrophe in Senior Care community.

It's almost predictable that results will show that a tragic combination of a virulent bug, poor administrative policies, inferior infrastructure, and deficient processes and procedures worked in synergy to escalate the virus' spread and its death toll.

Let regulators do what they do, but we can't afford to wait. The only way forward for our industry is to focus on what is in our power, including the changes that we can implement now to prevent another tragedy in the future.

After all, think about the same problem but from a very different perspective…

A public health or government official, city Mayors, Governors, or the President, must think about 'controlling the spread' and focus on the macro level. Steps they recommend to 'flatten the curve', like social distancing, contact tracing, wearing masks, etc. may be useful for solving the problem they are solving.

But our problem is a completely different one.

As an operator of a Senior Care community, I have the responsibility for the safety of 20 senior lives and the happiness of their families. It's like being the captain of a jet carrying 20 passengers coming in to land, with a Coronavirus storm raging around the airport.

Every day the news media is bombarding us with horrifying lightning and thunderbolt-like stories, visibility is zero, the air traffic control is giving unreliable directions, and my instrumentation dashboard is messed up. My passengers are panicking, their families down there are worried, my flight attendants are nervous, and I'm running low on fuel. I have no alternate landing sites, and despite all this, it's still my responsibility to bring in my plane and land safely. No one may applaud me for doing my job successfully. Some may even sue me for the work I do, and yet, I must succeed.

While Dr. Fauci, the President, the Governors or the Mayors may offer upbeat predictions while pointing to professional-looking PowerPoint slides until we all fall asleep, we are obliged to think for ourselves. It is incumbent upon us to think as the captains of our passenger jets in whom the passengers, their families and the community as a whole have vested trust in.

The Emerging Trust Deficit

The statistic that is keeping residents and their families up at night and eroding their faith in our communities is that 42% of US deaths due to Coronavirus are from just 0.6% of the population[22] (Figure 7). And, that 0.6% of the population was our residents, the people who entrusted themselves to our care.

This confirms that the senior care industry was ground-zero of this pandemic, a fact that is rapidly generating a trust deficit in the market that we serve. Whether this lack of trust will be a short term phenomenon or have lingering effects (economists call this hysteresis) is something only time will tell.

Unfortunately, we must all assume that the effects on our market will persist long after the cause is removed – perhaps by the mass availability of a Coronavirus vaccine. After all, history[24] tells us that long after vaccines were available for prior contagions, it took years for the entire population to become immune.

Even as biological immunity is unpredictable, likewise no one can predict psychological immunity from the fear and apprehension the deaths of so many in our care has generated.

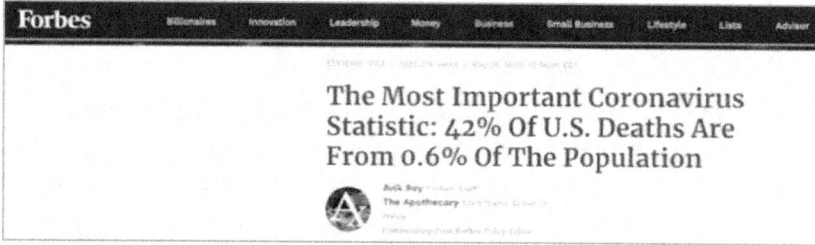

Figure 7 : Senior care industry was the ground-zero of Coronavirus

Rebuilding Trust

The sweeping effects of the pandemic on our industry and the resulting trust deficit among prospective residents and their families mean that we as an industry need to be proactive.

Regaining the trust of our customers is critical.

Yet, we will never succeed in rebuilding that trust if we don the cloak of "we were fully compliant with regulatory requirements and report fully and accurately to them"[18]. Instead, we have to recognize that no one was prepared for this catastrophe:

- Hospital systems were not prepared
- Regulators were not prepared
- Healthcare research & administrative institutions (CDC, CMS, CDSS, etc.) were not prepared

- Large and small nursing care and Senior Care communities were not prepared
- Seniors and their families were not prepared

The Coronavirus pandemic caught us all by surprise. The only thing we could do was react.

However, there is a light in all the darkness.

Now, that we have experience in dealing with the fallout from the virus' spread, we understand far more about not only where our previous approach to infection control and prevention was lacking, but also how we can proactively prevent and contain future outbreaks.

Goals vs Strategy vs Tactics vs Tools

The difference in these terms is of significance to winning this war against the pandemic for our senior citizens and thus regaining trust after the COVID-19 storm. Goals are the overarching objectives in war and strategy is a way of achieving those overarching objectives. Tactics are battlefield maneuvers to be employed on a day-to-day basis, while tools are the equipment or systems with which we implement a strategy.

Generally, all the recommendations coming from CDC are in the tools category (e.g. face masks, sneeze shields, disinfectants, etc.). The state oversight organizations (e.g. CDSS in California) are making the tools (recommended by CDC) available and are giving tactical guidelines and best practice recommendations. There are very few iron-clad 'must-do-else-get-cited' mandates.

What is missing until now (Summer 2020) is strategic thinking.

The reason why that is so important is that the perspective is different. The perspective of government institutions such as the CDC, as well as state oversight and licensing bodies is population care, whereas the perspective of the owner/operator/investor is that of the pilot with many passengers coming in to land in the storm.

For us (senior care community owners, operators, and investors), the strategy is important. For the most part, the only thing that even remotely sounds like a strategy is 'flatten the curve' or tactics like 'shelter-in-place', but we recognize them as reactive.

This book goes beyond the reactive.

It proposes a strategy that aims to neutralize the damaging effects of Coronavirus and other contagious diseases. By adopting this strategy, we can move into a proactive posture. We can come out of our bunkers and take the fight to this pandemic.

A New Way of Thinking

On June 8, McKinsey pointed out[17]:

"The pandemic has forced the adoption of new ways of working. Organizations must reimagine their work and the role of offices in creating safe, productive, and enjoyable jobs and lives for employees"

In the same way as offices and organizations are now required to adapt, this book focuses on what the Senior Care industry can do, without waiting for the long regulatory route to take shape, a choice that would leave our residents at risk[13].

Instead, we must focus immediately on strengthening the resistance of our Senior Care communities against the spread of all types of infections, such as MRSA, C-Diff, Influenza, Coronavirus, and the next virus that makes itself known.

That is why the "InfeXBloc™" operational architecture was developed.

Modeled after architectures that have already seen successful implementation in other industries, like commercial aviation and Information Technology data centers, InfeXBloc™ moves the Senior Care industry from the 'implicit-trust' approach to a 'proven-trust' (or 'zero-trust') infection security model.

In the implicit-trust model, everyone is 'safe' unless they exhibit 'unsafe' symptoms. Sadly, this is a model that led to the sweeping death toll of Coronavirus for our residents.

On the other hand, in the proven-trust model, everyone is 'unsafe' unless they establish their 'safe' credentials using an objective and repeatable process.

We will discuss in detail:

- underlying conceptual ideas, architectural designs, engineering, process and procedural suggestions that Senior Care communities can implement immediately
- proposals of various innovations like InfeXPASS™ (an RN certified designation of a person's health status), InfeXCON™ (a community's real-time risk designation), an 'InfeXBloc Scorecard™' system (to rate communities' implemented infection safety measures)
- how to adopt specific clinical protocols** to increase resistance to infection transmission while retaining the residential setting

** *it is important to note that Assisted Living community are licensed as non-clinical communities in most states. CDC has detailed recommendations[21] for infection control for clinical acute and non-cute care settings.*

Leveraging distributed architectures

The InfeXBloc™ operational architecture is a solution that leverages historical lessons that show that moving from a centralized to decentralized architectures produces better outcomes and improved resilience, including:

- When human governments moved from central control to distributed control (from monarchy to democracy), we empowered citizens to be free agents and take more responsibility. The result was an improved quality of life and a prosperous society.
- When computer architectures moved away from central control (as in mainframes) to distributed control (as in public clouds), increased processing power was leveraged. The result was that computing power multiplied many times and automation prospered.
- When planning architectures moved from central planning (as in the USSR) to decentralized planning (as in a market economy), we empowered free enterprise and independent decision making and dramatically improved economic output.
- When terrorism architectures moved away from central control (Al-Qaeda and its leader UBL) to distributed control (as in local terrorism cells), they became harder to track and more lethal. While the outcome for the civilized world was undesirable, the evil trade of terrorism prospered.
- For Senior Care, if we move from a centralized infection management architecture (of hospitals doing the work based on CDC guidance) to a distributed infection control architecture (like InfeXBloc™):

    - We will increase community empowerment.
    - An empowered community will take more responsibility resulting in better outcomes for seniors.
    - Regulators will gain an improved handle on the occurrence and propagation risk of infection.
    - We will increase the resilience of a community's overall healthcare infrastructure, in the face of future outbreaks (from Figure 8 to Figure 9). Keep in mind that experts say we are not done with Coronavirus yet and that even if a vaccine was developed tomorrow, another virus in the future is far more than just a possibility, and more likely a certainty!

In Japan, where the topography puts its population of 127 million in the pathway of earthquakes, landslides, and typhoons. Often, architects there, use sabo techniques[31] to slow down the velocity of water and debris flowing to prevent the overwhelming the downstream valley. We could use the sabo techniques to slow down the velocity of infectious senior residents flowing into the community hospitals and prevent them from getting overwhelmed, thus obviating the need to require economic lockdowns.

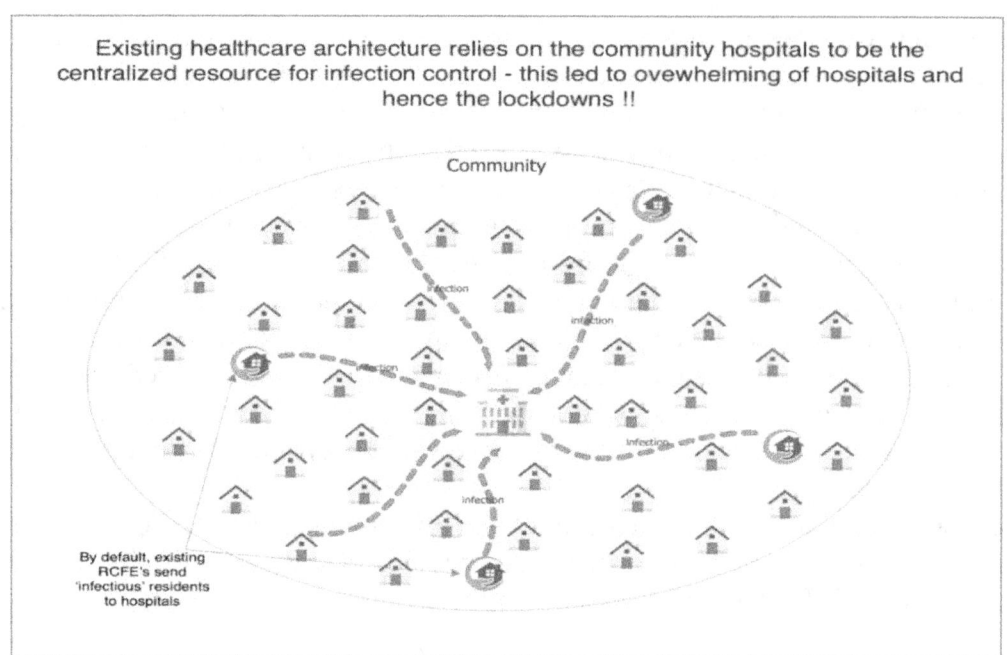

Figure 8 : Existing Senior care communities shift the infectious cases to hospitals

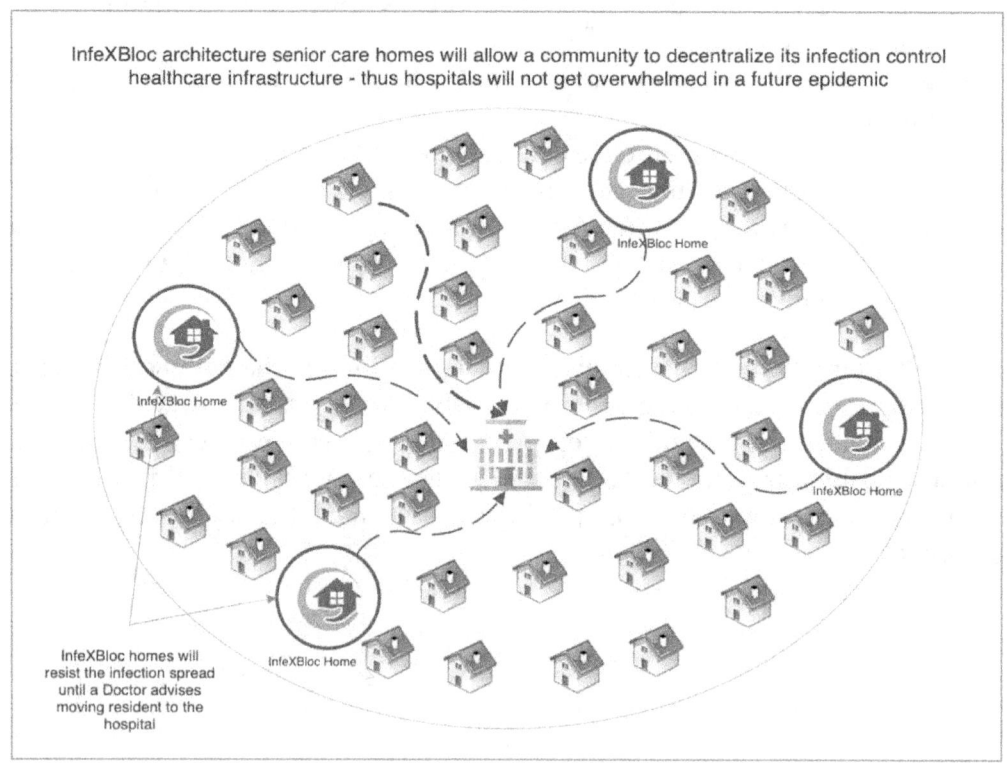

Figure 9 : InfeXBloc™ community will resist the infection spread

From fragile to anti-fragile

In his ground-breaking book 'Antifragile'[16], Nassim Taleb presents an extremely insightful hypothesis that architectures span a spectrum of Fragile → Resilient → Robust → Antifragile (Figure 10).

- **Fragile**
  - At risk of total failure / financial ruin

- **Resilient**
  - Takes damage, avoids total failure, recovers

- **Robust**
  - Absorbs uncertainty, repels blows, avoids damage

- **Antifragile**
  - responds to stress by mutating, maintains fitness for purpose
  - purpose and identity can change entirely

Figure 10: Nassim Taleb's fragility spectrum

The InfeXBloc™ operational architecture is a move towards developing anti-fragility. It aims to gain from the disorder unleashed by COVID-19.

When adopted, not only will it help Senior Care community resist further tsunamis that can overwhelm our community hospitals, but also improve the care these communities can offer to their senior residents.

Chapter 2: Lessons from the Past - from Airlines to Cybersecurity

On Sep 11, 2001, Al-Qaeda terrorists changed the prevalent paradigm in commercial aviation security, forcing a move from an 'implicit-trust security model' to a 'proven-trust model'.

Before the attack that changed the face of our nation, we could walk directly to the aircraft boarding gates to see off friends who were traveling or receive them at the gate. Before the advent of automatic baggage scans, our checked baggage was simply lined up next to the aircraft staircase and we would identify our suitcase before boarding.

The implicit assumption was that no passenger would carry a bomb – an assumption that was shattered by the suicide terrorists.

Since then, air travel around the world has never been the same. Proven-trust protocols have been implemented. These protocols are safer, but also dramatically more painful, expensive to implement. They significantly change the operational architecture (infrastructure, processes, protocols, tools, technologies, etc.) we once knew – a fact that is evidenced by the hardship experienced by travelers when dealing with the TSA. Yet globally, we have accepted the pain and expense because the assets we wish to protect (our own lives) are priceless.

In another domain, up until a few years ago, all enterprises had their own private, on-premise data centers. Cyber-security protocols were based on a notion of a 'castle and moat' – a strong perimeter defense called firewall(s).

This notion relied on the idea that what is outside the firewall is bad and whatever is inside the firewall is good, thus resulting in "whatever is inside can be trusted." This meant that software applications inside the enterprise could easily communicate with each other inside the trusted firewall ring.

The advent of public clouds changed this.

The paradigm switched from implicit-trust-based cyber-security to proven-trust, which once again led to pain for the security and network professionals within the enterprise. To transition to public clouds, proven-trust protocols had to be implemented.

We have relied on examples of Silicon Valley pioneers (Google, Amazon, Netflix, etc.) to communicate the need for proven-trust protocols to clients. New approaches[14] used by these pioneers in this domain are called containerization, micro-services, and micro-segmentation architectures that employ 'zero trust' as their core. This has significantly changed the operational architecture (infrastructure, processes, protocols, tools, technologies, etc.) that IT data center practitioners once knew. Once again, while these protocols are safer, they were also dramatically more painful and expensive to implement and significantly changed the infrastructure architecture and operational procedures. Yet globally, we have accepted the pain and expense because the assets we wish to protect (our enterprise data) are priceless.

Finally, in the late nineties, the internet led to the birth of e-commerce, a new channel for shopping. However, almost as soon as it took off, many publicized episodes of bankcard fraud had a crippling effect on the trust new consumers had on this channel.

Banks and e-commerce websites (eBay, Amazon, etc.) had to diligently re-invent identity verification protocols to ensure the innovation did not die prematurely, moving to a zero-trust model. Globally, we have accepted the pain and expense because the assets we wish to protect (our personal and financial data) are priceless.

Chapter 3: Foundations of Safety – Hazards, Controls, Swiss Cheese, and Risk

Let us unpack this non-trivial topic (Figure 11) to really understand risk and how better safety can be achieved.

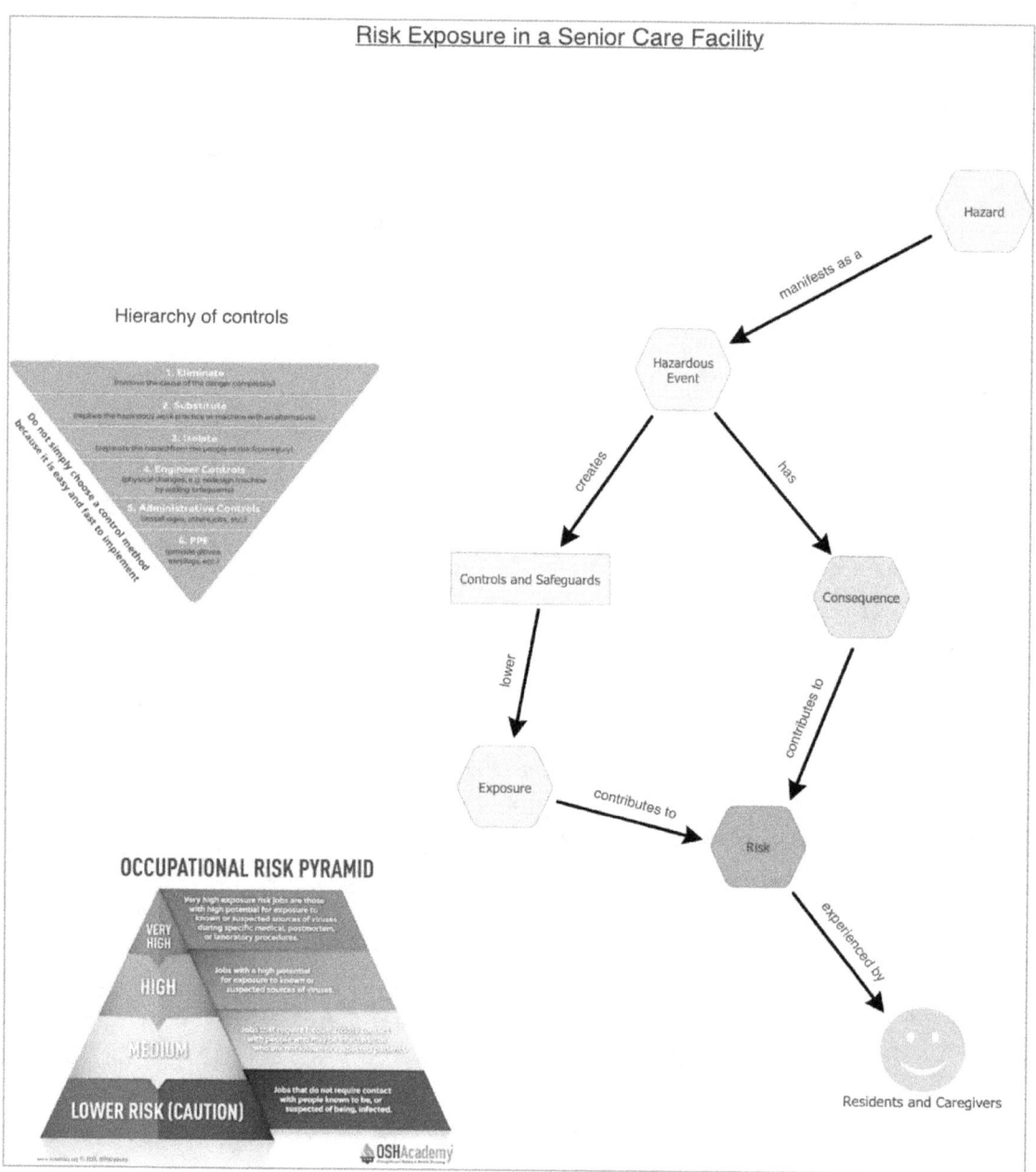

Figure 11: Understanding Risk

- A hazard is any agent that can cause harm or damage to humans, property, business, or the environment.

- A hazardous event is an instance of the hazard
- A consequence is the outcome of exposure to the hazardous event.
- Risk is defined as the probability that exposure to a hazard will lead to a negative consequence, or more simply, a hazard poses no risk if there is no exposure to that hazard.
- A safeguard or control is that which creates a space between us (humans/property/our business) and the hazardous event. It protects humans/property/businesses from the shock energy of the hazardous event.

For example, live electricity is a great hazard. In our homes, in every room, we are surrounded with live 220 V electricity flowing through all the walls. However, there are very strong controls and safeguards between us and that hazard, like insulation of the wires, UL certified switches, appliances with insulation, etc. that create a safe space between us and the hazard. The safety created is enough that we sleep peacefully on our beds and lose awareness that we are surrounded with a deadly hazard.

Risk can be seen as the product of the severity of consequence times the probability of exposure. Consequently, risk assessment always starts with hazard identification.

Three important features depicted in the graphic (Figure 11) tell an important part of this story:
- Predictable -vs- Unpredictable
- The occupational risk pyramid
- The hierarchy of controls

Predictable vs Unpredictable

The credit for the deep insights in this section is attributed to Dr. Todd Conklin and his book "Workplace Fatalities – Failure to Predict"[35].

Most sets of industrial events in our business domain are predictable in nature. Hence, if a large enough data set of historical events is studied and signals recognized, we could predict the next occurrence with reasonable confidence. If we could predict, then we could work on prevention approaches. However, some events are complete outliers and of those, some have very high consequence. These are called Black Swan events. A Black Swan[36] event is easy to simplify after it happens, but remarkably hard to notice before it happens. These events are non-linear and non-predictive. The only thing we can do is build capacity in the system to minimize the consequences of such events.

Fatalities are not normal events. They happen as outliers to the way normal work happens. A fatality is not a logical ending of a bad safety program. Hienrich's accident pyramid does not apply to such high consequence events that are outliers.

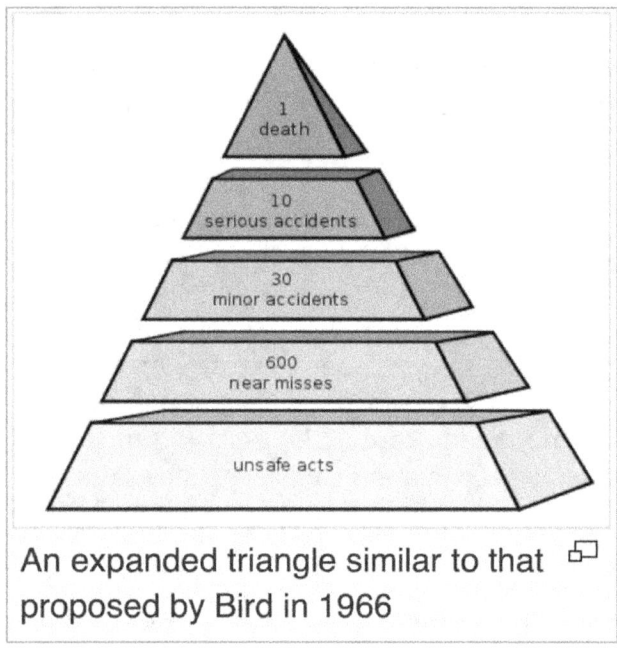

Figure 12: Hienrich's Accident Pyramid

If you look at the pandemic like a normal failure because of a safety lapse, worst still the logical climbing of the accident pyramid (Figure 12), then you are likely to focus on that event alone and you will miss the entire opportunity for a deeper learning. You will work harder on the lower-level events believing that the same approaches that solve the lower-level events will solve the catastrophic events, you will just create wasted motion. Your organization will get better at low-level events, you may have fewer falls, but you will not get more reliable around the high consequence events. In other words, you want to shift the thinking of your organization from solving for the failure to prevent the last event to solving for more effective matching of controls and safeguards for the next event discussion. The body of knowledge around catastrophic events (like this pandemic) is purposefully different than the body of knowledge around lower consequence safety events. These Black Swan events are not simple events that we could prevent. These events are complex failures that happen on many levels of the organization and simply defy the ability to be predicted by the organization.

The Coronavirus pandemic was one such event. The last such event was a century ago. Systems built in the last hundred years had no capacity to minimize the consequences of it. That covered a wide variety of systems – transportation systems, healthcare systems, financial systems, aviation systems only to name a few. With the absence of capacity, it is not surprising that the impact of this pandemic has been so catastrophic. Because these Black Swan events are not predictable, not only must we implement robust safety programs to address prevention issues, but we must also expand our thinking to work on a program to implement controls and safeguards that provide recovery when such events happen. For example, in 2020, we would not want to drive a car with no seat belts. The chances of you getting in a wreck are slim, but the recovery that the seat belts provide in case a wreck happens, is priceless. This is particularly true if your family is riding with you in that car.

For the Senior Care business ecosystem, no one can predict when the next such event may happen. For such events, we must manage the event probability as well as event recovery in parallel. There may be no way to predict the entry of a Coronavirus infection (or other infections) that can be deadly to our vulnerable senior residents, hence we must have a robust recovery program. Given that, it is incumbent upon us to build capacity in our system to make sure that when this happens next time, we have the capacity to prevent uncontrolled harm.

The Occupational Risk Pyramid

The occupational risk pyramid grades different occupations based on the exposure the worker has to a different level of hazard (e.g. an IT worker working remotely using Zoom has a far lower exposure that a utility lineman working on high tension transmission wires). Depicted in Figure 11, OSHA classifies occupations into 4 categories based on the expected exposure to hazard Very High, High, Medium, and Low. For healthcare workers, OSHA[37] classifies as follows:

Very High Exposure Risk

Very high exposure risk jobs are those with high potential for exposure to known or suspected sources of COVID-19 during specific medical, postmortem, or laboratory procedures. Workers in this category include:

- Healthcare workers (e.g., doctors, nurses, dentists, paramedics, emergency medical technicians) performing aerosol-generating procedures (e.g., intubation, cough induction procedures, bronchoscopies, some dental procedures, and exams, or invasive specimen collection) on known or suspected COVID-19 patients.
- Healthcare or laboratory personnel collecting or handling specimens from known or suspected COVID-19 patients (e.g., manipulating cultures from known or suspected COVID-19 patients).
- Morgue workers performing autopsies, which generally involve aerosol-generating procedures, on the bodies of people who are known to have, or suspected of having, COVID-19 at the time of their death.

High Exposure Risk

High exposure risk jobs are those with high potential for exposure to known or suspected sources of COVID-19. Workers in this category include:

- Healthcare delivery and support staff (e.g., doctors, nurses, and other hospital staff who must enter patients' rooms) are exposed to known or suspected COVID-19 patients. (Note: when such workers perform aerosol-generating procedures, their exposure risk level becomes *very high*.)
- Medical transport workers (e.g., ambulance vehicle operators) moving known or suspected COVID-19 patients in enclosed vehicles.
- Mortuary workers involved in preparing (e.g., for burial or cremation) the bodies of people who are known to have, or suspected of having, COVID-19 at the time of their death.

Medium Exposure Risk

Medium exposure risk jobs include those that require
frequent and/or close contact with (i.e., within 6 feet of) people who may be infected with SARS-CoV-2, but who are not known or suspected COVID-19 patients. In areas without ongoing community transmission, workers in this risk group may have frequent contact with travelers who may return from international locations with widespread COVID-19 transmission. In areas where there *is* ongoing community transmission, workers in this category may have contact with the general public (e.g., schools, high-population-density work environments, some high-volume retail settings).

Lower Exposure Risk (Caution)

Lower exposure risk (caution) jobs are those that do not require contact with people known to be or suspected of being, infected with SARS-CoV-2 nor frequent close contact with (i.e., within 6 feet of) the general public. Workers in this category have minimal occupational contact with the public and other coworkers.

It is reasonable for us to see how caregivers in Senior Care communities will fall into the Medium – Very high risk spectrum. As for our healthy residents they may get classified in the Medium to High-risk spectrum. However, since our residents are in the 65+ age bracket and often have several underlying health conditions that lower the strength of their immune system, they represent a group with higher vulnerability (Figure 13) . Consequently, it is imperative to assume that our residents are in the high to very high category.

COVID-19 Hospitalization and Death by Age

Rate ratios compared to 18-29 year olds

	Hospitalization[1]	Death[2]
0-4 years	4x lower	9x lower
5-17 years	9x lower	16x lower
18-29 years	Comparison Group	Comparison Group
30-39 years	2x higher	4x higher
40-49 years	3x higher	10x higher
50-64 years	4x higher	30x higher
65-74 years	5x higher	90x higher
75-84 years	8x higher	220x higher
85+ years	13x higher	630x higher

Source: CDC
https://www.cdc.gov/coronavirus/2019-ncov/covid-data/investigations-discovery/hospitalization-death-by-age.html

100 – 600 times more deadly

Figure 13: Pandemic's Asymmetrical Impact on Seniors

The Hierarchy of Controls

In safety literature, the hierarchy of controls is an inverted triangle (Figure 14) and it grades controls and safeguards from the most effective to the least effective from top to bottom.

- Elimination — Physically remove the hazard
- Substitution — Replace the hazard with a lower consequence substitute
- Isolation controls — Isolate people from the hazard
- Engineering controls — Engineering methods to distance people from hazard
- Administrative controls — Change the way people work
- PPE — Protect the worker with PPE

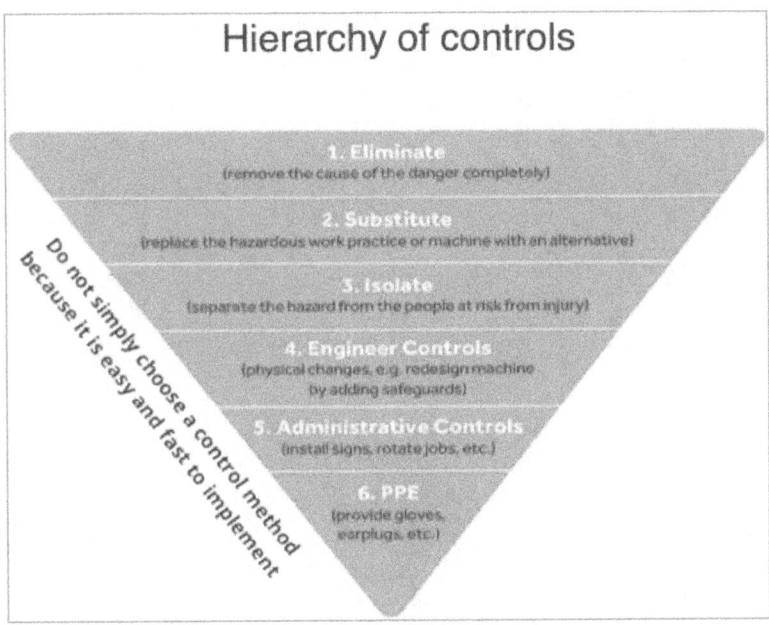

Figure 14: Hierarchy of Controls

It is interesting to note that the PPE (personal protective equipment) is the least effective control to be employed because it is the last line of defense between the hazard and the caregiver or healthy resident.

Businesses and workplaces often use a combination of controls classified at different levels to make the location safe. The more that we can incorporate controls and safeguards of the higher categories, the lower the risk of exposure to hazards. In the section titled "Classifying controls and Safeguards in InfeXBloc™" we will categorize our recommendations.

The Swiss Cheese Model

In 2000, James Reason described a model[40] of how failure can propagate in a complex system by using the metaphor of layers of swiss cheese. Figure 15 shows multiple layers of barriers that exist between a hazardous event and our residents/ caregivers/ staff/ community/ business. Each barrier can be perceived as a safeguard/procedure/protocol/engineering control/administrative control/PPE layer. The model describes how each layer is not bullet-proof all the times. Each has its own weaknesses that appear and disappear momentarily. A hole in the swiss cheese layer can represent a weakness that can manifest momentarily. Almost all the times, the holes in all the layers do not align and thus there is a separation maintained between the hazardous event and our residents/caregivers/staff/community/business. This way, most of the time the energy of the hazardous event cannot propagate through.

However, on an unpredictable occasion, the holes in multiple layers (weaknesses in different layers of the barriers) can align and when that happens the energy of the hazardous event can propagate through and harm our residents/caregivers/staff/community/business. This model of how failure can propagate in complex systems and lead to uncontrolled harm has been observed in multiple noted examples like the sinking of the Titanic, the Three Mile Island nuclear accident, the Challenger Space Shuttle accident, the Shuttle Columbia disaster, September 9-11 terrorist attacks, and Hurricane Katrina.

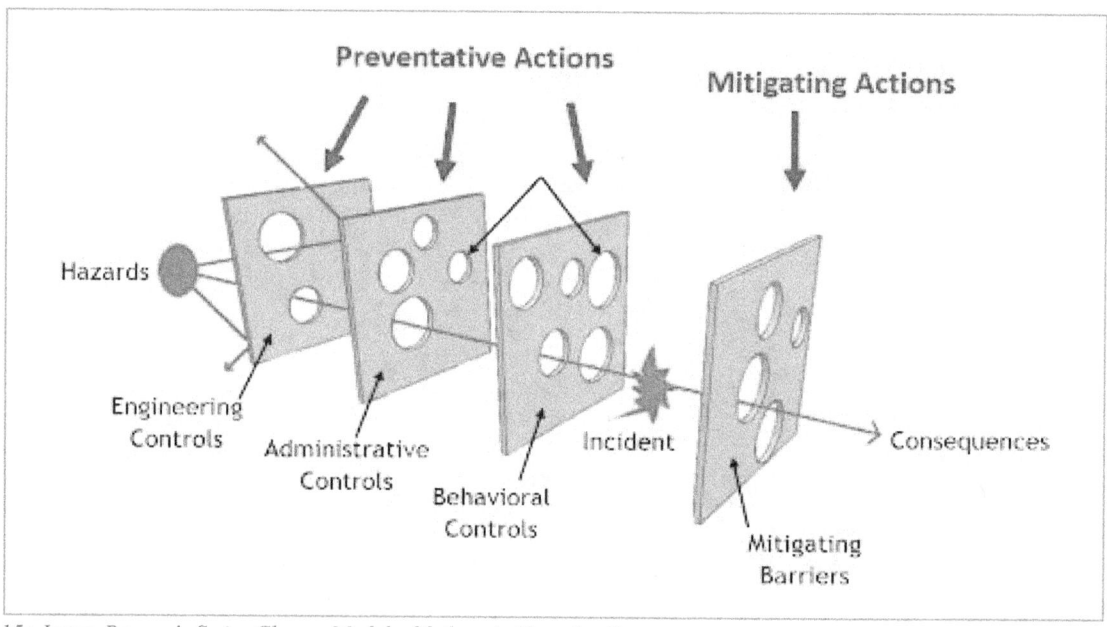

Figure 15: James Reason's Swiss Cheese Model of failure in Complex Systems

There are many reasons why weaknesses can momentarily appear in these barriers and weaknesses in multiple barriers that can align unpredictably and allow hazards to come in contact with the caregiver/resident/staff/community/business and causes harm.

Weaknesses, that can be temporal, can be divided into two categories:

- Active failures: are unsafe acts committed by caregivers/professionals who are in direct contact with residents, equipment, or the system. These have a direct and typically short-lived effect on the integrity of the defenses.

- Latent conditions: are hidden in the design and working of the system, environment, or equipment. They lie dormant in the system until they combine with an active failure to create an opportunity for harm to occur.

Active failures can take a variety of forms like slips, lapses, mistakes, and violations. Latent conditions can come into play due to ineffective training, inadequate supervision, ineffective communications, inadequate staffing, ineffective equipment, unworkable procedures, poor design of devices, communities, equipment, or supplies.

While latent conditions can be improved, active failures cannot be entirely eliminated. There is no solution to these weaknesses that appear momentarily in different layers. By keeping on building and improving the multiple layers of barriers, we lower the probability of the hazard being able to cause harm, thus lowering the risk.

Safety as Capacity

I have a personal connection with this topic of safety. I grew up in the 60s in a little town called Bhilai in India. It is a town built around a massive integrated steel mill. I remember seeing signage like Figure 16 throughout the town, noticing signs in the mills when we would go on field trips (the Coke Ovens, the Blast Furnace, the Plate mill, the Rail mill, etc.), with messages like "Safety Awareness Week", "248 days without an accident" or "Congratulations to Blast Furnace Team! Celebrating 100% on safety inspection" etc. That was my first initiation into the importance of safety measures. Many decades later, on 9th October 2018, my childhood friend, Uday Pandey, fell victim to an industrial accident[32] at the same plant.

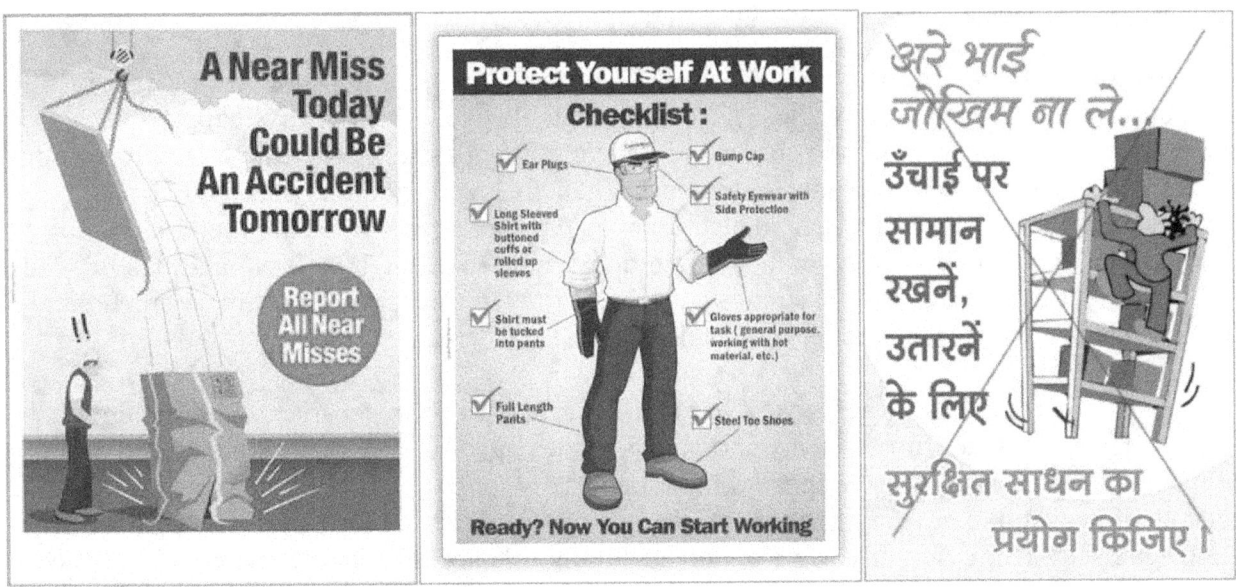

Figure 16: Safety signage in my childhood town

Safety is a feeling. Technically it is defined as a dynamic non-event. It cannot be measured directly. Safety is not the absence of accidents, but the presence of capacity[31]. That notion of capacity in this context is interesting. While often we use that term capacity to indicate a physical property of an object (e.g. a 5-gallon bucket), here we use it to refer to a system's property that allows that system to absorb the uncertainty of an accident.

Several examples are quite illustrative:
- When the building and safety department mandates earthquake code compliance, they are creating capacity in the structure to deal with the uncertainty of seismic shaking. Compliance with this code requires extra design, engineering, materials, and construction effort and a significant extra cost. But when an earthquake happens, the structure has the capacity to deal with it without causing uncontrolled harm.
- During the non-fire season, the department of fire must diligently implement activities like dry brush clearance, deadwood removal in forests, training of firefighters, developing equipment and infrastructure like air tankers, their fire-retardant supplies, staging airports, etc. If these capacity-building activities are adequately funded and executed in years before a fire ravages a certain section of California, then the system has the capacity to deal with a fire without it causing uncontrolled harm.
- In Silicon Valley are some of the giants of the digital economy (e.g. Google, Amazon, eBay, Netflix, etc.). In a short period, they have significantly altered the composition of economic activity. When you rely on cloud-based computer systems to carry out billions of dollars of business 24X7, you must think hard about disaster preparedness to deal with the uncertainty of emergent events. Netflix has invested years and a very large budget with a continuously improving effort to build capacity to deal with such uncertainty. That program is called Chaos Engineering and some of the products out of this program (called Chaos Monkey simulations) have been open-sourced.

In the Senior Care domain, accidents could be falls leading to injury to residents or a case of infection entering the community, etc. These unpredictable events will always happen. Developing safety, then is not their absence, but developing a capacity to deal with them without leading to catastrophic and unwanted outcomes. When analyzed from this perspective, it becomes clear that Senior Care as an industry lacked the capacity to deal with the virulent bug (Coronavirus). Once it entered several communities, it burned through their populations like the dry brush as we experience every summer with forest fires in California. It is not so much that people made bad choices, but people had bad choices.

It is easy to understand that when you have to build capacity, it is expensive, takes diligent well-directed effort, and takes time, when you don't have the capacity, coping with the effects of unpredictable hazards is really expensive and takes a very long time (not to mention the loss of precious life). Just like buying insurance is a hedge against financial risk, building capacity is a hedge against systemic risk. If you never had an automobile accident where the fault was yours, you may be inclined to feel that your insurance premium payments were an unnecessary burden, but one such unpredictable event and your view changes forever.

Capacity building, is a deliberate, well planned, and continuously executed activity. Regaining trust after this Covid-19 storm and fostering the feeling of safety will be a capacity-building activity. Most importantly, as in the case of insurance, capacity must be built before the risk materializes.

InfeXBloc™ is an operational architecture for a Senior Care community that will build a capacity to absorb the uncertainty of a pandemic, epidemic, local outbreak, or just a random infection. It will make the community pandemic resistant. Moving Senior Care communities to be InfeXBloc™ enabled will then be a capacity-building activity.

HFACS

Our industry is 'high touch', it is light on service automation and primarily delivers its services by way of human rendered care, hence, the occurrence of human error is unavoidable. Sometimes this can combine with other weaknesses in the senior care ecosystem and produce severe undesirable outcomes.

The Human Factors Analysis and Classification System[38] (HFACS) is a general human error framework originally developed and tested within the U.S. military as a tool for investigating and analyzing the human causes of aviation accidents. Based on Reason's (1990) model of latent and active failures, HFACS addresses human error at all levels of the system, including the condition of aircrew and organizational factors.

The HFACS framework was used to analyze human error data associated with aircrew-related commercial aviation accidents that occurred between January 1990 and December 1996 using database records maintained by the NTSB and the FAA.

Investigators were able to reliably accommodate all the human causal factors associated with the commercial aviation accidents examined in this study using the HFACS system. In addition, the classification of data using HFACS highlighted several critical safety issues in need of intervention research.

These results demonstrate that the HFACS framework can be a viable tool for use within the civil aviation arena. Developed originally in the military and aviation industries, these methodologies have been used by numerous fortune 500 companies including many well-renowned healthcare organizations. These innovative tools and methods are also espoused by many accrediting agencies and patient safety organizations within the healthcare industry.

InfeXBloc™ will pioneer the application of HFACS methodologies to the Senior Care industry.

Chapter 4: Hazard Identification

One of the "root causes" of workplace injuries, illnesses, and incidents is the failure to identify or recognize hazards that are present, or that could have been anticipated. A critical element of any effective safety and health program is a proactive, ongoing process to identify and assess such hazards. A detailed guideline[34] for this activity is specified by OSHA.

Senior Care is a complex ecosystem

The operational ecosystem of a Senior Care Community (called RCFE in California), as depicted in Figure 17, is complex. It's worth noting that almost all external entities that come in contact with these communities are in multiples (many pharmacies, many doctors, many hospitals, etc.), and they interact with the Senior Care community multiple times every day.

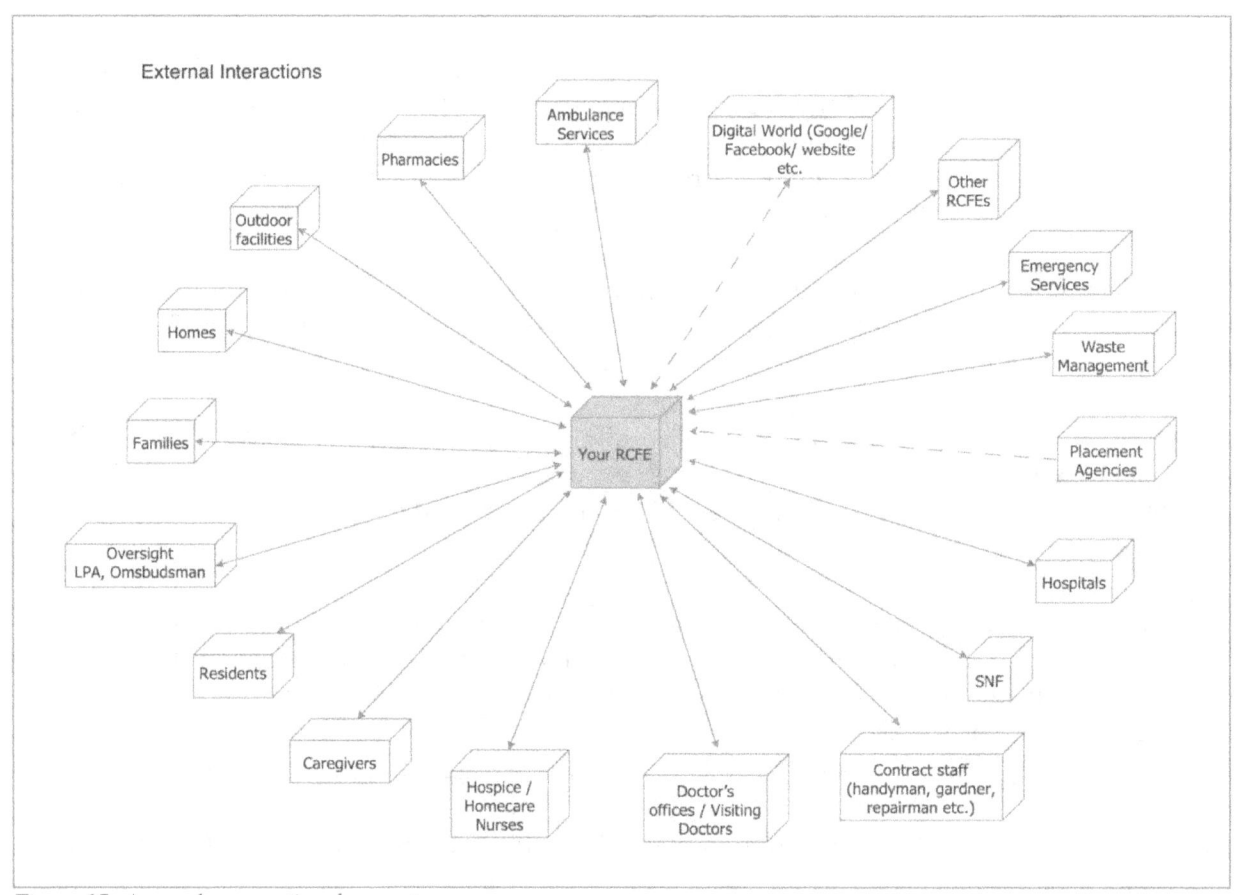

Figure 17: A complex operational ecosystem

This implies that the attack surface area (a terminology from the cybersecurity domain - the size and shape of the zone that exposes vulnerability) that communities must be concerned with is therefore very large.

While some industries can boast of the automatic benefits of remote working, Senior Care communities will continue to be a hi-touch industry. While there will be opportunities to use remote examination via 'telehealth-visits', the bulk of caregiving will remain hi-touch, requiring physical contact.

If we dig deeper to understand our community's level of exposure, we find that we can think of it in three parts:

- From the outside-in
- When the bug is already inside
- Transmission pathways
    - Via surface contact
    - Via aerial pathway

Each of the above exposure categories can result in an infection in a once healthy senior.

From outside

Every interaction with the outside world represents an infection transmission vector – a pathway along which infection can travel. In Figure 17, only the dotted lines represent interfaces that are not involved in possible infection transmission.

The number of ways in which infection can come from outside is:

$$(number\ of\ residents)\ x\ (number\ of\ visitation\ events\ from\ outside)$$

This grows geometrically as the bed capacity increases.

When the bug is inside

To go deeper, Figure 18 represents the interactions between the insiders. On the inside, we have two types of actors:
- human (residents, caregivers, visiting professionals, staff, contract workers, family members, etc.).
- non-human (care equipment like wheelchairs and walkers, cleaning equipment, faucets, doorknobs, etc., which once contaminated with a bacteria or virus can lead to spread).

Every interaction represents another infection transmission vector and like before, each entity is in multiples (many residents, many caregivers, many ADL activities, many visitors, many professionals, many pieces of equipment, many door knobs, many faucets, etc.). Inside the Senior Care community, the attack surface area grows exponentially.

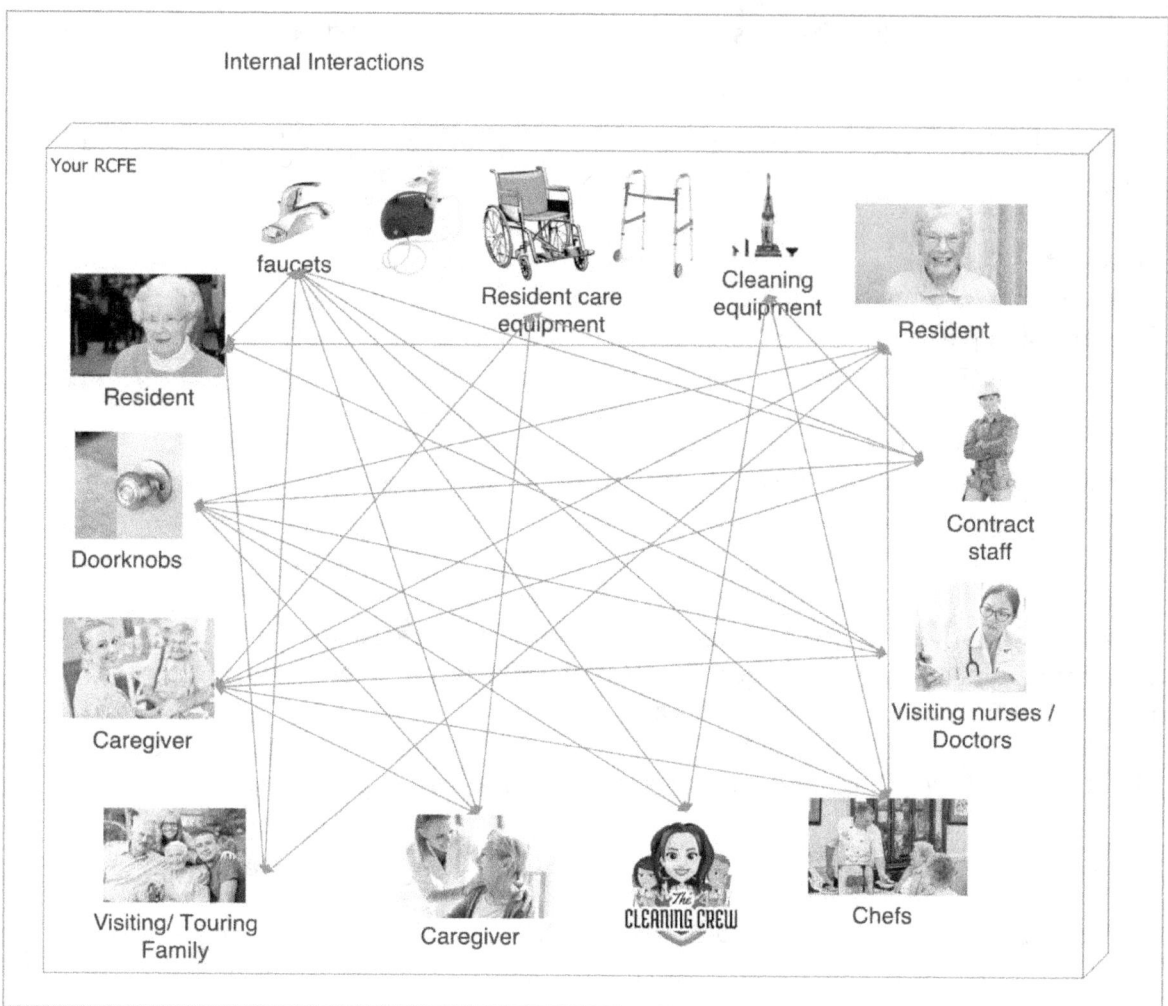

Figure 18: The complexity multiplies on the inside

The aerial pathway

In an eye-opening simulation[6] (Figure 19) of infection spread, the aftermath of an infectious person coughing in a grocery store aisle was presented.

In this time-lapse, we see the droplet- cloud spread rate via the aerial pathway. In this case, no contact disinfection methods (disinfectant sprays, wiping surfaces, UV lights, etc.) may be effective.

The issue is further compounded by the fact that in closed spaces, like in a Senior Care community, the HVAC system, which is traditionally not designed to disinfect, recirculates air. Theoretically, this makes the attack surface area hyper large and any human actor can be the source, with anyone in the vicinity becoming a target.

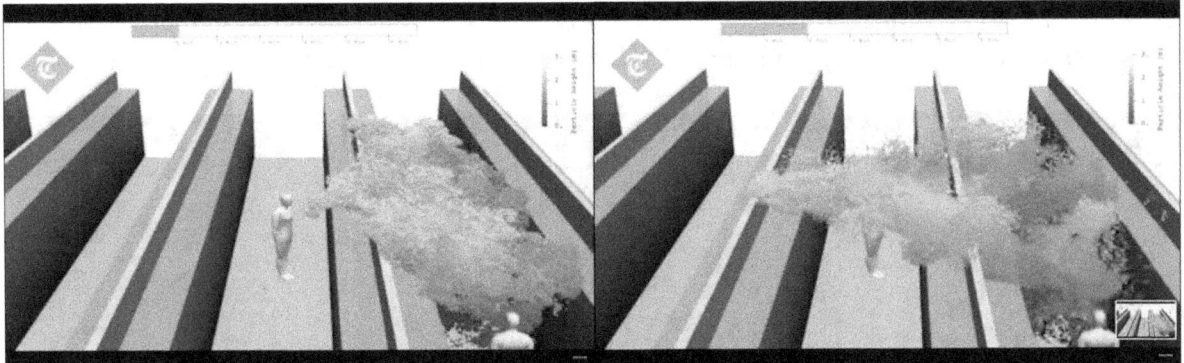

Figure 19: The aerial route

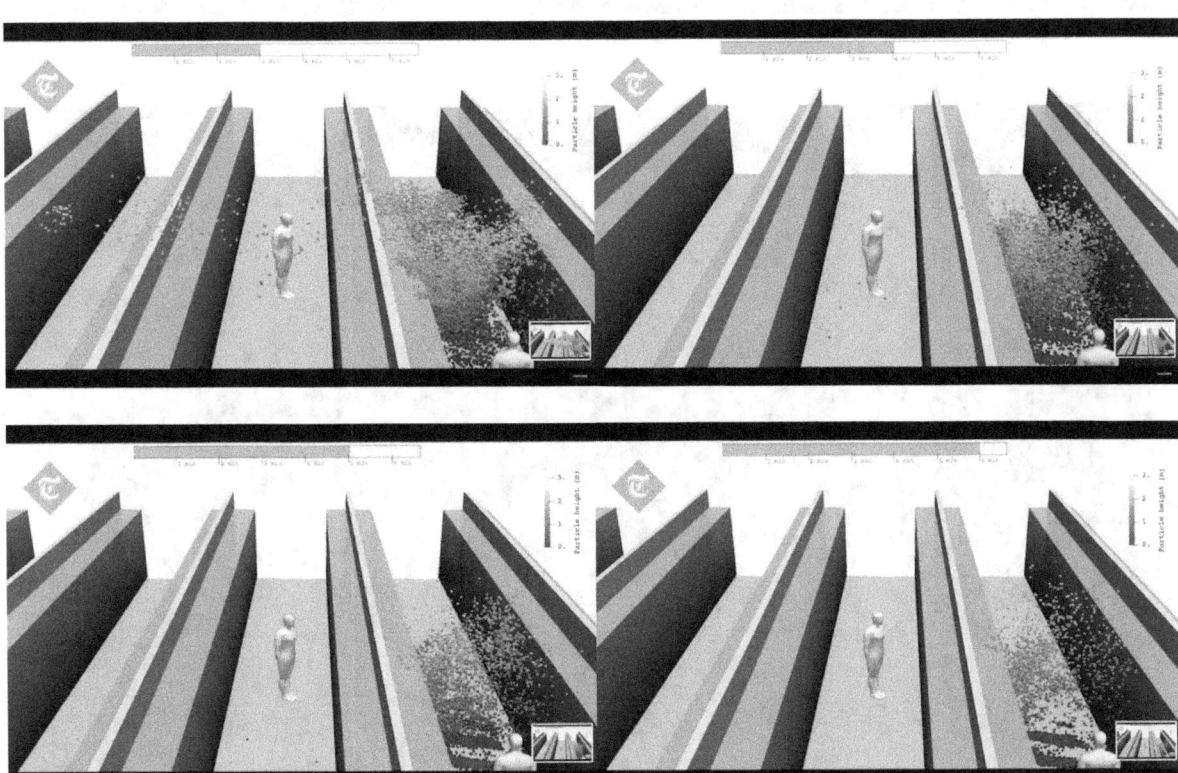

Another study in Japan (NHK) published a 'micro-droplet' infection transmission mechanism report[7]. Figures 20 and 21 depict the pictures from a high-speed infrared camera after a sneeze.

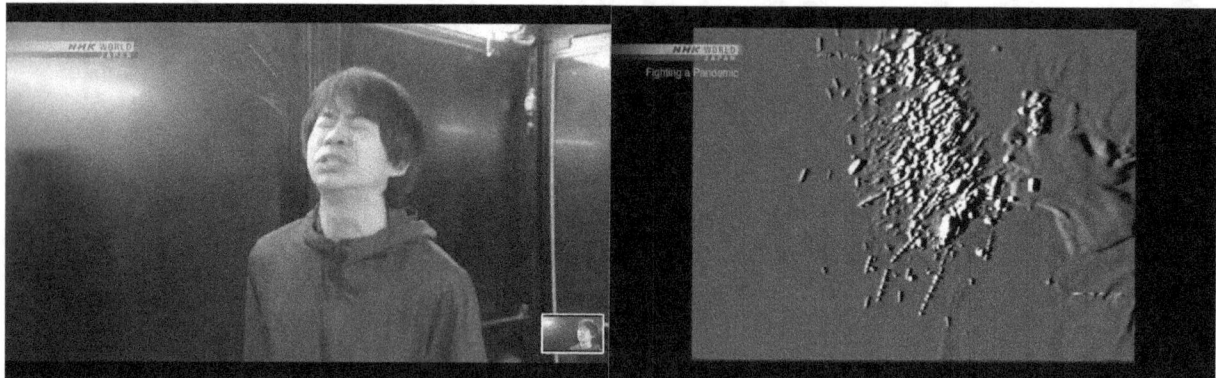

Figure 20: Man sneezing

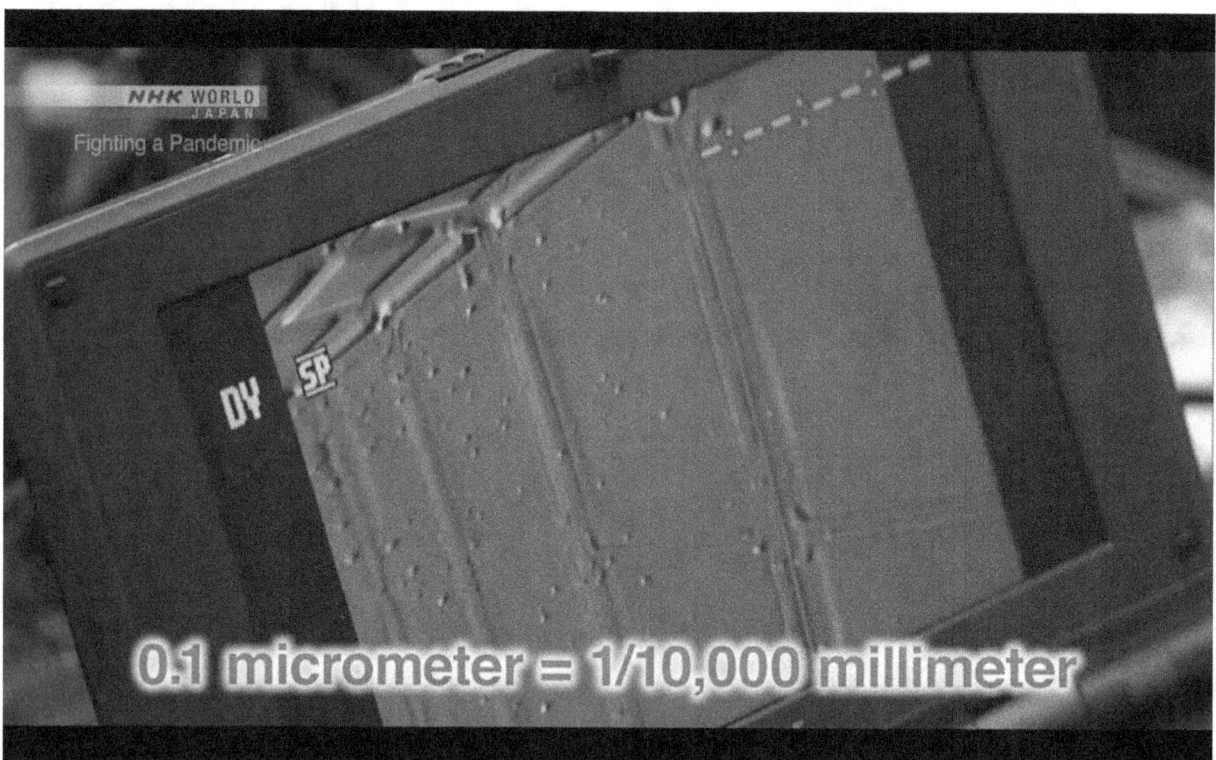

Figure 21: Micro-droplets linger on for a long time

The latest headlines from WHO[26] claim that data exists that Coronavirus is airborne (Figure 22). While we do not have much data about this aerial infection spread, it suffices to say that this dramatically increases the attack surface area needing defense.

Figure 22: Is Coronavirus Airborne?

Telemetry of the spread

One example of telemetry is how scientists track the movement of whales in ocean documentaries. Telemetry can also be used to track the spread of infectious viruses and bacteria.

Using these methods, if one were to track the sequence of:

- door handles touched to enter the resident room,
- the equipment touched (walkers, wheelchairs, breathing oxygen tubes, CPAP masks, etc.),
- the body contact during caregiving events (incontinence care, toileting, bathing, tooth brushing, etc.),
- meals delivery (food plates, bowls, delivery presentation, milk pouring, etc.) as well as post-meal cleanup activity,

we could theoretically arrive at the detailed telemetry of the infection spread.

An eye-opening (and scary) video[8], compiled by CNN, showed a black light simulation (Figure 23) of a dinner table setting and how quickly and completely germs can spread in a short time.

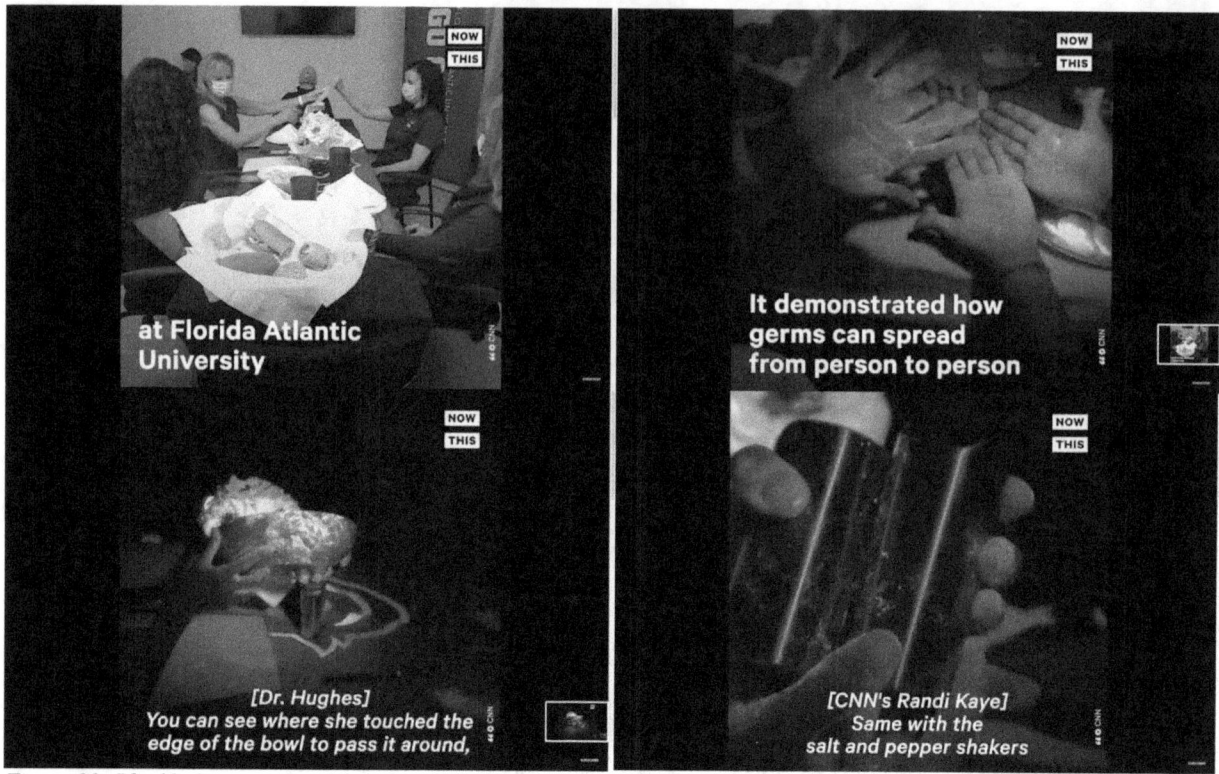

Figure 23: Blacklight simulation of spread telemetry

This is not new knowledge

Surprisingly, the huge attack surface area of germs and their spread telemetry not only existed but were assessed well before Coronavirus and have been highlighted in the GAO report[1,2] (Figure 25).

However, before Coronavirus, no one attempted to quantify the level at which MRSA, C-Diff, Influenza, and other diseases had ravaged senior living communities, simply because these other infectious diseases did not have a high fatality rate. The appearance of Coronavirus, a highly virulent bug exposed the chink in our armor.

The statistics in Los Angeles County (Figure 24) are eye-opening.

Cumulative and Active Cases by County

Figure 1: Graph of Cumulative Cases in RCFEs by County*

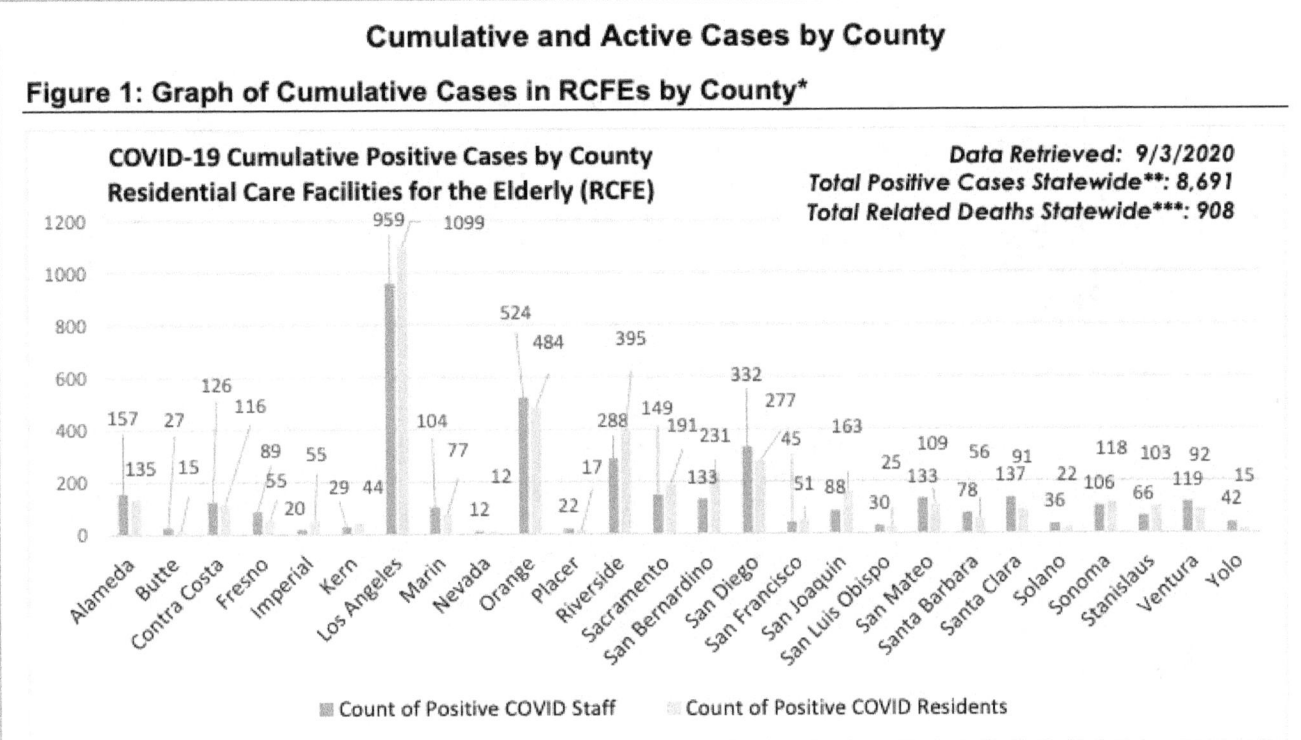

Figure 24: Los Angeles County (source CDSS)[20]

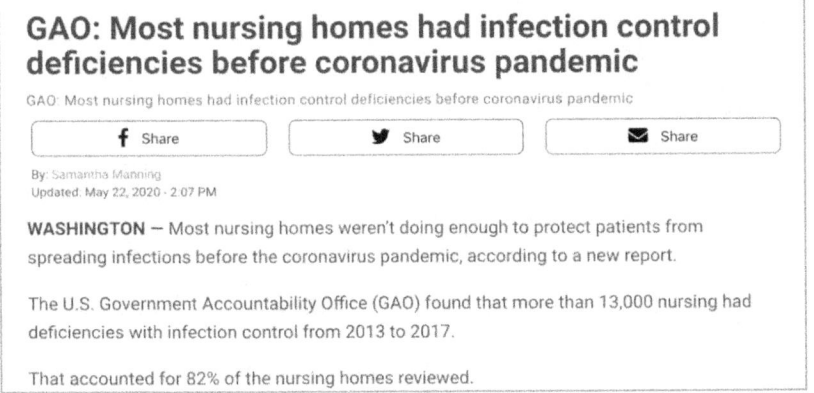

> "This did seem to be both widespread and persistent across the time period we looked at," said John Dicken, director for health care issues at GAO. "There were examples of staff who may have been doing direct care with residents but had not been doing effective handwashing in between residents. There was staff that were coughing or had fevers and were providing direct care."
>
>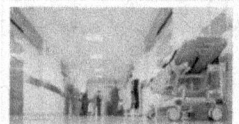
> SPONSORED CONTENT
> COVID-19 and Healthcare Risks: Urgent Resources for Urgent Times
> By Coverys
>
> In other cases, the investigation found that some facilities weren't doing enough to isolate infectious patients.
>
> "There were some residents that may have been mixed including some that were exposed or had some kind of infection," Dicken said. "One with a staph infection that was sharing bathrooms with other residents."
>
> >>>RELATED: State releases COVID-19 data for nursing homes, long term care facilities
>
> The report said Congress wanted this investigation done because of the threat to nursing home patients from COVID-19.
>
> "These have been a long-term issue and so the current environment really reinforces the need to focus on these types of infection control measures," Dicken said.
>
> There is ongoing work happening to look at how nursing homes are handling infections during the pandemic and how the federal government is enforcing regulations regarding infection control at the facilities.
>
> In a statement, a spokesperson for the Centers for Medicare & Medicaid Services (CMS) said:
>
> "CMS is committed to protecting the health and safety of our nation's seniors living in nursing homes. As the GAO described, insufficient infection prevention and control is frequently cited as a deficiency in long term care facilities. CMS has used this data to strengthen federal infection control and prevention regulations and policies. Both before and during the ongoing coronavirus disease 2019 (COVID-19) pandemic, CMS has provided nursing homes with resources to assist their efforts at combating infectious disease. CMS will continue to use every tool at our disposal to ensure nursing home residents are protected."

Figure 25: GAO Report

The 800-pound gorilla in our living room

In summary, given:

- the magnitude of the infection transmission issue that resulted in thousands of senior lives lost,
- the overwhelming attack surface area that we must secure. The more the number of beds, the more caregivers needed and the more non-caregiving staff needed, resulting in exponential growth of the infection attack surface area. (This should not be a relief to smaller 6-bed communities in California, who have been spared from the negative media blitz by the DSS statisticians.),

- the urgency of the fix, we cannot wait for years for a solution to present itself organically. Our customers, their senior parents, regulators, and society in general, absolutely everyone expects better (not to mention the trail attorneys),
- the mandatory preparedness that would be expected in the aftermath (Coronavirus may revisit us in the subsequent years),
- the regulatory oversight that will certainly increase,
- and the 'silver tsunami' which is just a few years away,

How should we move forward?

Complex systems are gnarly!

Complex Systems is indeed a complex science. While simplifying it may seem futile, we will attempt to do just that, in relation to the Coronavirus threat.

Most of us think of cause and effect as a linear process and we tend to draw it 'left to right' using bubbles and arrows. However, in complex systems, circular causality, feedback loops, time delays, exponential escalation, or decays are the norm. The result is that causes and their effects can be very non-linear and widely separated in space and time. The more interconnected the systems are the more the ripples travel. Societies are classic examples of complex ecosystems.

One of the diagramming techniques used in this science is the causal loop diagram (CLD). These are very intuitive to read and comprehend. A CLD for the impact of Coronavirus on our society appeared in a Lancet article[19] (Figure 26).

Below, some simple notations are used:

- arrows point "A impact B"
- a '+' sign at the end of the arrow means A and B move in the same direction, but a '-' sign indicates opposite movement
- parallel bars imply a time delay
- sometimes loops are formed which can result in accelerating or dampening behavior in the system (observe the red loop). This is often referred to as circular causality and can cause runaway effects

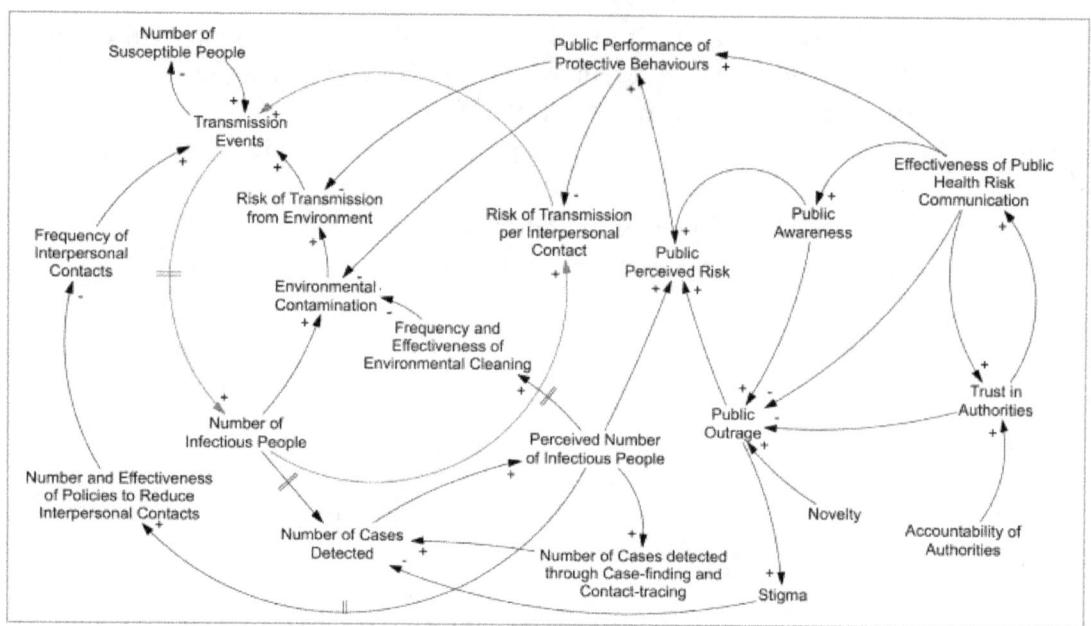

Figure 26: An example causal loop diagram for the COVID-19 threat

As the Figure 26 makes obvious, causes and their effects are not so straightforward. Even though techniques (called systems science) to analyze and predict the behaviors exist, approaching in that manner is clearly out of scope for this book. So, we will sacrifice that scientific rigor, and approach this empirically.

Chapter 5: Overcoming this challenge with InfeXBloc™

InfeXBloc™ will help us overcome the deficiencies exposed by this pandemic. Let us unpack this.

Statics -vs- Dynamics

The physical features of an InfeXBloc™ enabled community will generally implement most of the recommendations in the report "Strategies for Safer Senior Living Communities" (from the American Institute of Architects)[43]. However, the InfeXBloc™ operational architecture goes well beyond this and tackles process, procedures, protocols, tactics and training – all aimed at creating pandemic resistance. One easy way to distinguish between a building architecture of a community and its operational architecture would be to think of the distinction between statics and dynamics (by dynamics I am not implying ideas like shape shifting buildings). What gets built before business operations start is what I am grouping in the 'statics of a community' whereas, what happens after the community commences operations is the 'dynamics of the community'. Both of these aspects have strong implications on infection spread. This dynamics in a community manifests infinite opportunity for infection spread (as detailed in the chapter 'Hazard Identification'). The InfeXBloc™ operational architecture goes inside the dynamic life of this active business (of a Senior Care Community) to uncover and address those attack vectors that cause the infection spread.

Conceptual underpinnings of InfeXBloc™

History tells us that a medieval castle that relied only on its moat to keep the enemy out, lost when the enemy was airborne or already inside (compromised insiders). In our context, this translates to accepting the uncomfortable notion that one or more of our resident is already infected (thus infection is already inside), ready to take down our communities and our healthy seniors.

Introducing friction

In a highly compromised domain, the only way to thwart the spread of the enemy is to introduce friction against its movement. This is a best practice in several domains:

- multiple concentric check points in a military installation prevent the lateral movement of a threat.
- multiple identity check points in the commercial aviation domain we implemented after September 11, 2001, attacks.
- multiple authentication and authorization checks are implemented in cloud-native IT architectures.

While in real life, completely sterile environments may only be found in cleanrooms used for surgery, NASA labs, or pharmaceutical manufacturing, the only way to deal with a highly compromised domain is by introducing friction along the transmission path. This concept is already employed universally:

- air conditioning systems use HEPA filters to snag air-polluting particles
- automobile engines use oil and fuel filters

In our own effort to resist infection spread, we already leverage several steps to introduce friction in the pathway of infection spread:

- using alcohol-based disinfectants
- washing hands
- PPEs (gloves, facemasks, face shields, gowns at appropriate intervals)

InfeXBloc™ architecture adopts this same paradigm change to the senior care industry to enhance safety and care.

Provable and Repeatable process

In the aftermath of 9-11, in the aviation industry, every visitor or passenger approaching the airport was by default designated unsafe. Then, through a series of provable and repeatable safety checks, he was designated safe while inside the perimeter. This was achieved by implementing checkpoints set up at multiple concentric perimeters within the airports – a practice inspired by a military doctrine called defense-in-depth as contrasted to castle-and-moat. Anytime the passenger exited the perimeter, his security disposition had to be reset to back to unsafe.

With the advent of public clouds, in the cybersecurity industry, key paradigms were shifted. Authentication and authorization systems switched from:
- 'default allow unless explicitly denied access' to 'default-deny unless explicitly allowed'.
- firewall rules for virus scan software systems switched from 'blacklisted websites' to 'whitelisted websites'.

Implicit Trust policy

Our operating model before March 2020 (the one which failed to protect our residents with the advent of Coronavirus) was implicit-trust-based. Everyone was 'safe' unless they proved otherwise. This meant that we could focus most of our energies on actual caregiving. Community infrastructure was more directed to caregiving needs, e.g., fall prevention features, like grab bars in corridors and bathrooms, non-slippery ambulatory surfaces, clutter-free rooms, etc.

Proven Trust policy

In the proven-trust policy, we reject the comfort of the assumption that it is automatically safe inside the Senior Care community and instead embrace the danger of the assumption that the bug being already present inside. Thus, everyone is 'unsafe' unless proven otherwise.

For years, we acknowledged that Influenza, MERS, C-Diff, Pneumonia, and other diseases are infectious and often appear in our communities. Yet, Coronavirus, its high infectiousness and fatality rate have gotten everyone's attention and shown us that assuming our communities are safe spaces is no longer an option.

As a consequence, Senior Care community must now focus on caregiving as well as stopping infection spread and must adopt a new safety architecture that addresses the inherently large attack surface area.

A proven-trust safety architecture would strongly resist the lateral movement of the threat. It would consist of a combination of two distinct approaches working together to keep residents, staff, and visitors safe:
- Implement strong perimeter (Figure 27)
- Implement maximum transmission friction (Figure 28)

A strong community perimeter

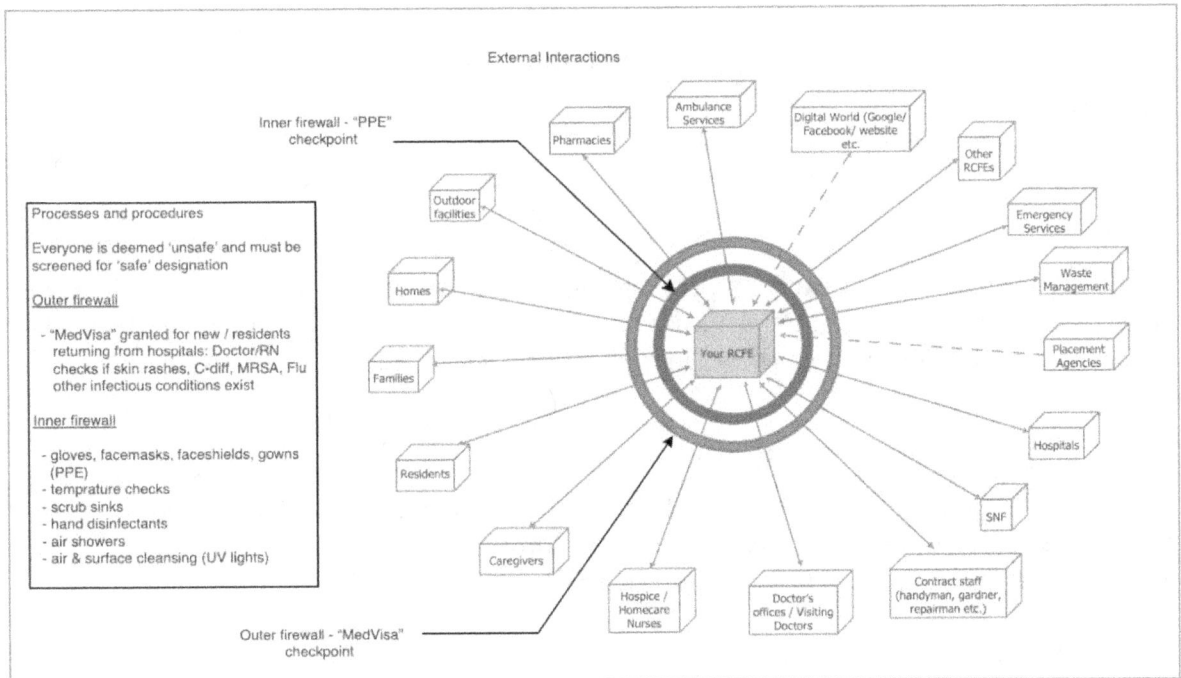

Figure 27: Strong perimeter

The above introduces a notion of "InfeXPASS™" which functions as a medical clearance that implies the entrant into a Senior Care community is safe. This may manifest in two ways.

- A licensed practitioner (Doctor, PA, RN) screens a new resident/returning resident from a hospital stay and certifies him as infection-free. A lighter version of it will be for family or guest visitors who may closely interact with the residents (red ring in Figure 27).
- Both the above will be accompanied by an inner firewall (purple ring in Figure 27).

Resident room perimeter

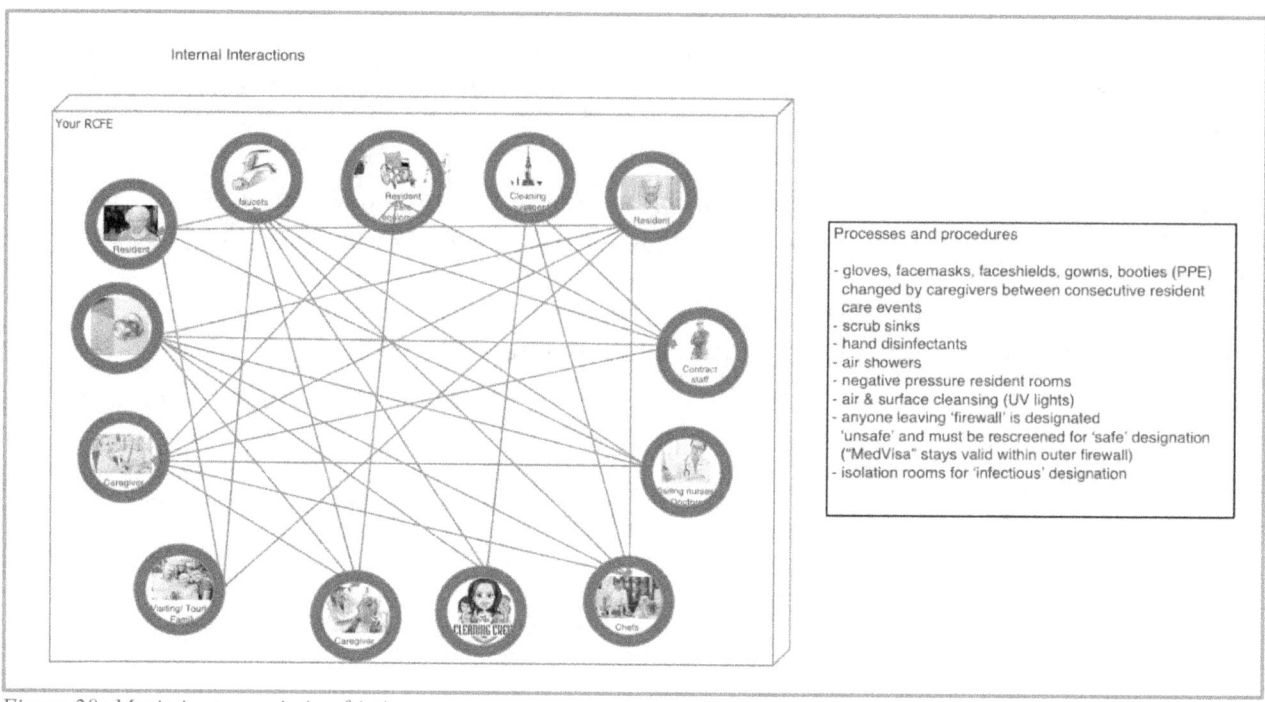

Figure 28: Maximize transmission friction

Figure 28 illustrates the idea that each resident's room must be designed to defend itself in order to maximize resistance to infection transmission within the community. This is accomplished by adopting a host of procedures that work in synergy to block cross-transmission inside the community.

An operational Senior Care community represents a, ecosystem of human (with residents, caregivers, visiting families, maintenance staff, etc.) and non-human actors (caregiving equipment, wheelchairs, doorknobs, etc.). When each contact between these actors is sandwiched between disinfecting steps, we greatly increase the resistance for infection transmission.

This will be achieved in several important ways:

- Consumables (disinfectants, gloves, face masks, face shields, protective gowns, etc.)
- Equipment (touch-free doors, touch-free faucets, UV lights, negative air pressure HVAC, etc.)

- Processes (single entrance gate, resident room doors that can require caregivers to swipe access cards, check if a caregiver has her face mask and gloves on, etc.)
- Procedures (create a robust audit trail of events to establish adherence to protocol)

Defining 'Proven trust'

Overall the 'proven-trust' framework will combine both the controls (Figure 29) by erecting a strong perimeter to guard against the virus entrance, while at the same time maximizing friction of transmission within the community:

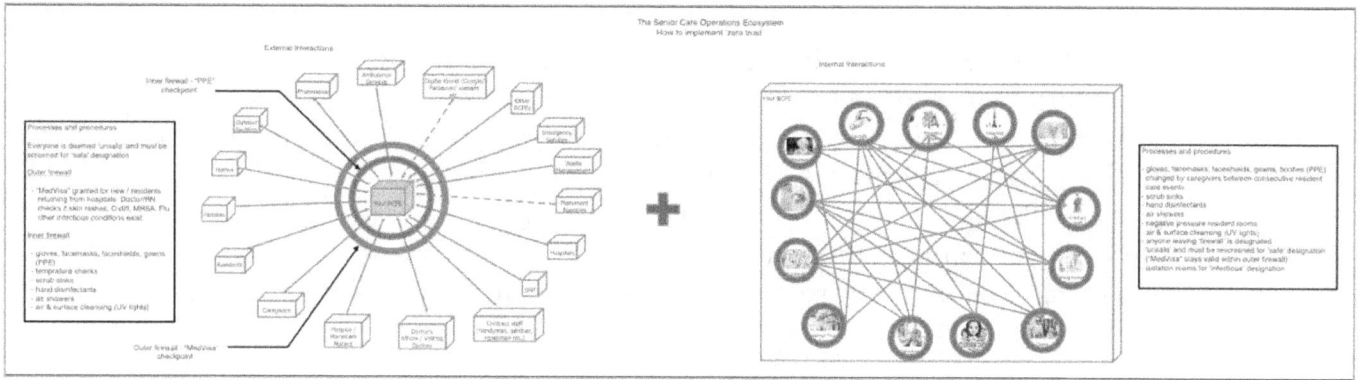

Figure 29: Implementing 'proven trust'

Please use zoom capabilities to view Figure 29 details.

Implementation of InfeXBloc™ - Leveraging technology

The implementation of InfeXBloc™ will involve various technological and process elements:

1. Unified entrance complex
2. Strong physical perimeter fence
3. Access ID key card for each entrant
4. 'InfeXPASS™' that becomes part of the key
5. Enforcement of PPE usage (facemasks, face guards, sneeze guards, etc.)
6. Automated sliding doors for resident rooms and touch-free faucets, touch-free doors, faucets, lights, toilet flushes, bidets, soap-disinfectant dispensers
7. Deploying UV lights to disinfect
8. Negative pressure HVAC
9. Digital touch-free visitor log
10. Designate 'InfeXCON™' status for the community (like DoD designates a DEFCON status when they want a military installation(s) to operate at a heightened alert)
11. Interlinking of the key card, the InfeXPASS™ status, the automated sliding doors security system, and the InfeXCON™ designation to control access to each critical resource (resident rooms)
12. Deploying the security principle of 'least privilege'

13. Video recording of all events in the community
14. Correlate the resident billing to the community InfeXCON™ status
15. Deploying Isolation Rooms
16. Deploying voice activation (Alexa, Siri, etc.)
17. Deploying fall alarms
18. Deploy a scoring system – InfeXBloc Scorecard™

Using a unified entrance complex

A singular entrance complex will be used for the following purposes:

- Controlling access, validating authentication and authorization
- Providing a Nurse to grant or deny 'InfeXPASS™'
- Providing for change of street clothes into community provided scrubs at the start of shift (and vice-versa after the end of shift)
- Utilizing thermal cameras for temperature sensing
- Receiving of deliveries from suppliers
- Providing temporary exit-passes and infection-controlled breakroom for caregivers

Using an access-id card for each entrant

Each entrant will be provided a magnetic stripe key card/fob key. This card will contain data points like:

- User's identification
- InfeXPASS™ status
- Authorization privileges that implement the least-privilege pattern
- Community InfeXCON™ designation that this access card is valid for

Using an 'InfeXPASS™' encrypted access-id

An InfeXPASS™ will function as a medical certificate attesting to the health of the access cardholder, which can be any of the following:

- granted or denied by a Nurse at the entrance (for residents, caregivers, volunteers, activity staff, etc.).
- self-certified by visiting Doctors, RNs, LVNs (grouped as 'credentialed professionals').
- employer-certified for licensed contract staff or employees of delivery companies.

The Key card is surrendered when the holder leaves the community premises. If a holder of the access card develops unsafe medical symptoms, his access is revoked, and he will be immediately escorted outside the entrance complex.

Using enforcement of PPE utilization

Every resident room will have a facial scanner outside the door to scan for the N-95 face mask, gloves, other PPE required, and allow or disallow the opening of the sliding door when the key card is swiped.

Using automated sliding doors for resident rooms

Automatic doors will provide a touch-free mechanism for entering the micro-perimeter of the resident's room.

Using equipment to resist aerial transmission

Several technologies will help:

- Negative pressure HVAC systems with high air changes per hour (OSHPD standard[5] for isolation rooms is 12 ACH).
- Anterooms that allow caregivers to discard PPE after a care event for an 'infectious' resident.
- Airflow is directed from the ceiling to the resident's bed to exhaust through the vent. The general recommendations for directional airflow is from common areas → corridors → anterooms → resident room → bathroom → exhaust
- Returning exhaust from a resident room should not mix with clean air going to the room.
- Air scrubbing/cleaning within the room (e.g. SAM400 from Scientific Air Management)
- There are recommendations for optimum humidity maintenance to thwart virus life

Defining an 'InfeXCON™' status for the community

The community will have 4 operational InfeXCON™ status, which changes based on current conditions:

Green

- No one is 'infectious';
- room doors can stay closed; because PPE usage is still enforced
- meals are served in Dining Hall;
- Activities are ongoing in 'Great Room'
- Unified entrance complex operates to screen inbound guests/relatives/professionals/staff
- UVC lighting does disinfection routine sweeps

Brown

- One resident (or more residents, but the count is below the x% threshold – this threshold can be decided by the community management) is 'infectious'
- their rooms are quarantined; Negative HVAC is on; their meals are served in their rooms
- their caregivers are on heightened alert; PPE usage is strongly enforced.
- other residents use common areas; dining areas; activities are on for them.
- group activities can be streamed live for quarantined residents.
- video messaging on between healthy and quarantined residents.

Yellow

- More than threshold (x%) residents are 'infectious'.
- their rooms are quarantined; Negative HVAC is on; their meals are served in rooms.
- all caregivers are on heightened alert; PPE usage is strongly enforced.
- common areas, dining areas are closed; activities are suspended.
- video messaging on between healthy and quarantined residents.

Red

- One or more residents have tested COVID-19 positive (or other high severity infection)
- all rooms are quarantined; Negative HVAC is on; their meals are served in rooms.
- all caregivers are on heightened alert; PPE usage is strongly enforced.
- common areas, dining areas are closed; activities are suspended.
- video messaging on between healthy and quarantined residents.

InfeXCON™ is a transient status and can be changed in either direction based on a licensed practitioner's decision. The strength of protocol definitions may change as we deal with different types of infections.

Integrated authentication and authorization

- Interlinking key card, InfeXPASS™ status, automated sliding doors security systems, and InfeXCON™ designation control access to each critical resource (resident rooms, laundry rooms, visitation rooms, medicine cabinets, etc.).
- Deploying the security principle of 'least privilege' – this is the physical equivalent of 'need to know' in the information world. For example, a caregiver need not have access to the central medicine storage, which only the Medtech can access.

The community will have 'black boxes'

- Video cameras will be installed in each room and common areas (indoors and outdoors) and will record events in real-time. This will be designated as the VDR.
- The audio feed from all resident rooms and common areas will be recorded on a separate track. This will be designated as the ADR.
- Data events will be recorded from each data point in the community. This will be designated as the EDR.

These three 'black boxes' for the community, when correlated together, will paint a complete digital picture of the lead up to a observation event and its context at the point of reference. The data from these black boxes is encrypted and is only decipherable using a decryption key which will only be available for authorized personnel. Conceptually this is identical to black-boxes in commercial aircraft which provide forensic intelligence in a crash investigation. This technology has now been adopted by the automobile insurance industry also.

Correlate the resident billing to the community InfeXCON™ status

- The pricing structure may factor in the InfeXCON™ status as follows:
    - Base pricing assumes InfeXCON™ status is Green.
    - Incremental pricing may apply when InfeXCON™ designation is turned Brown, Yellow or Red.
    - Every morning a text message is sent to the resident's family member's phone to provide status updates. A new update will also be sent each time the community's InfeXCON™ status is escalated or downgraded.

Implementing change management

As complex as the Senior Care community ecosystem is, the InfeXBloc™ architecture itself is a complex proposition with many moving parts:

- Infrastructure
- Equipment
- Consumables
- Processes
- Procedures and protocols
- Humans

What is also clear is that InfeXBloc™ is a dynamic architecture (unlike a static architecture drawing).

As the architecture is implemented in communities, corrections and improvements will occur. As newer tools technologies and tactics become available, they will be incorporated. This is why we propose an organized and agile approach to managing these changes.

We propose:

- Defining a Stakeholder council comprising of operators, resident council members, administrators, caregivers, families, LPA, and Ombudsman.
- Maintaining a list of feature backlog by the administrator.
- Voting for prioritization of items on this backlog by stakeholders.
- Stabilizing on a quarterly cadence for the deployment of changes.
- Providing training on changes being deployed next quarter for all staff.
- Informing stakeholders when new changes are deployed.
- Soliciting feedback.
- Communicating upcoming changes to all stakeholders in the monthly report.

Implementing the InfeXBloc Scorecard™

Peter Drucker is often credited with a key management quote - *"If you can't measure it, you can't improve it."*

InfeXBloc Scorecard™ is a first proposal for developing an objective measurement system that can be used to assess infection control effectiveness so that it can be continuously improved. It will provide a balanced scorecard that incorporates multiple assessment criteria, including:

- Ingress control
- PPE preparedness
- Transmission resistance processes
- Disinfection protocols
- Isolation rooms
- Family-friendly access protocols

Implications of deploying InfeXBloc™ architecture

When the new paradigm of 'proven trust' security is adopted, actors involved will feel a significant impact. Let's take a look at that impact:

On community owners, operators and investors

The adoption of InfeXBloc™ architecture can be expected to deliver:

- a demonstrably safer community for senior residents and their families with a quantifiable proof point for the assertion
- a sound defense in the event of arising legal liability
- a certifiable audit that creates a strong viable evidentiary trail
- a InfeXSIM™simulation proof point to help justify the investment
- real-time visibility of the InfeXCON™

- a balanced scorecard (InfeXBloc Scorecard™) to achieve quarterly ratings to brag on
- a codified measurement mechanism to assess the value of a business

On architects & designers

The physical architecture must now pay attention to the implementation of the following:

- A strong perimeter entrance gate, entrance temperature check station, caregiver changing room (from street clothes to community cleaned scrubs, donning of PPEs, the deposit of cell phones, etc.)
- Design of rooms for 'infection containment' (negative pressure HVAC, touch-free door, touch-free faucets, private baths as far as possible, anterooms, the ability for caregivers to discard biohazardous waste, air scrubbing equipment, etc.)
- Possible design of sunroom – as this has disinfectant qualities and is beneficial for seniors
- Hands-free sliding room doors to minimize contact surfaces
- Hands-free faucets that automatically activate/deactivate to minimize contact surfaces
- Shower handles, toilet flush handles, doorbells should be cleansed/disinfected regularly
- Pressure-indicator outside of rooms will indicate if the room is under negative or positive pressure so that the caregivers can determine the course of entry
- Scrubbing stations in rooms as well as for a collection of rooms
- UVC lights for room disinfection

Several of these features have been included in the AIA report[43].

On the process architecture

The process design should pay attention to the implementation of the following:

- Verification/validation/medical check for granting of 'InfeXPASS™'
- Mandatory handwashing between every caregiving event
- Residents with an infectious sickness will not leave their rooms and will be provided with meals in the room
- No bags permitted past the outer firewall
- Community should
    - not allow street footwear, rather will provide disinfected house shoes for everyone except non-caregivers who must wear work boots as part of OSHA compliance. These will be provided booties.
- Groceries, vegetables, meats, fruits, supplies, bags, and similar items will be cleaned and disinfected before storage
- Schedule rooms/common areas will be vacant for one hour per day for UVC disinfection
- Laundry will be done once a day separately for each resident to avoid cross-contamination amongst residents' laundry

On the equipment

The use of senior care equipment will need to factor in the following:

- Wheelchairs, walkers, canes, gurneys, blood pressure monitors, thermometers, medicine carts, nurse's iPad, and other care equipment must be cleaned and disinfected
- Stairs, banisters, elevator components, furniture, and other community fixtures must be cleaned and disinfected
- Books in the library should be cleaned and disinfected

On the PPE

The community should now
- pay attention to the supplies of and the usage of PPE and must ensure that PPE is changed before and after every care-giving event with an 'infectious' resident
- consider storage of PPE (e.g. face masks, gowns, gloves, etc.) near the resident rooms (perhaps in anterooms) rather than just a central storage
- dynamic inventory of PPE should be published on a Safety Dashboard on the InfeXBloc™ Mobile App. Such a publication will allow the stakeholders to be informed in real time, in case this inventory starts experiencing shortage

On caregiver health

Caregiving creates undeniable stress on the frontline staff (in Safety and Resilience engineering circles the term 'sharp edge' implies the same). The community should pay attention to the health of its caregivers in the following ways:

- Physical health
    - Caregivers need to be careful with their health, declaring the presence of coughs, colds, fevers. If present, taking leave until they are healthy is important.
- Emotional health
    - Employee Assistance Programs will be available for caregivers to deal with 'caregiver stress' or other causes of stress.
    - Workload rebalancing will be used to deal with extra work when one or more of the residents in a caregiver's rotation is designated 'infectious'.
    - A caregiver reporting 'sick' or 'infectious' must withdraw from active caregiving tasks.

On resident's family members

Resident families should be educated about the shared responsibility of placing their beloved senior in an InfeXBloc™ community in the following ways:

- Visiting family members must obtain InfeXPASS™ screening, wear appropriate PPE, booties, etc.

- Physical contact with residents will only be across plexiglass dividers or 'hug-screens' if the community is not in Green status.
- Give a scoring card (InfeXBloc Scorecard™) for resident families to score a community.
- Encourage virtual visits if the community is not in Green status.
- Weekly 'State-of-Mom' video report will be posted on the website which will include her medication journal, care journal, etc. (this is based on Mom's HIPAA permissions)
- Family members can have authenticated access to "Mom's Page" on the community website.
- All "Mom's Treasures" (physical and digital) will be part of a farewell package delivered to the family after Mom's death.

On placement agencies

Placement agencies may:

- Use the InfeXBloc Scorecard™ to gauge the suitability of a community for their clients.
- Encourage prospective residents to use a virtual 3D tour to preview a community. These will be magic carpet ride tours beyond the current Matterport video tours and will be available long before the community is built.
- Follow visitor protocol during open-house tours.

On residents and the care-service, they receive

Residents should expect:

- Some restrictions to mobility when they are diagnosed with 'infectious' diseases unless the Doctor designates them as needing isolation, in which case they will be relocated to 'isolation' rooms (if such a room is available, otherwise they will be transferred to a hospital).
- To use face masks when interacting with other residents.
- To be outside of their room when the UVC light/Robotic disinfecting will be performed.
- A stronger cleaning and disinfection routine.
- To enjoy more connectedness via virtual visits.
- More personalization.
- Meetings with family members will adhere to 'social distancing' norms until normal operations resume.

On healthcare providers

Doctors, Nurses, and other health professionals:

- Can self-certify their 'InfeXPASS™'.
- Should follow the PPE protocols.

- Should encourage virtual health visits.

On non-caregiving staff

Chefs, handymen, equipment maintenance staff, hairdressers, delivery staff, and other non-caregiving staff:

- Should enter only via 'entrance complex'.
- Must sign a declaration to obtain 'InfeXPASS™' on site.
- Should avoid resident contact unless essential.

On oversight - regulators, inspection (LPA), Ombudsman

Regulators, Inspection agents, Ombudsman and similar individuals will:

- Be enabled for virtual visitation and virtual inspection.
- Have access to monthly 'State-of-InfeXBloc™ community' video reports.
- Be able to use conference rooms for personnel interviews, audit reviews, etc.

On volunteers

Volunteers must sign a declaration to secure 'InfeXPASS™' on site.

On activity staff

Activity staff must:

- Sign a declaration to secure 'InfeXPASS™' on site.
- Avoid contact with residents.

On delivery staff

The delivery staff will:

- Have their company certify their 'InfeXPASS™'.
- Minimize contact with residents.

On the cost of care

It is important to recognize the cost implications of implementing a paradigm change. After 9-11, commercial aviation security switched from 'implicit-trust' (every flyer is safe unless they proved unsafe) to 'proven-trust' (every flyer is unsafe unless they proved safe) and this had huge cost implications:

- Airport architectures had to be redesigned.
- Security checkpoints, X-ray machines, baggage screenings, safety perimeters, traffic patterns around airports had to be redesigned.
- Process architecture had to be fully redesigned.
- Total travel duration planning had to be redone for airline travelers.
- TSA had to hire a brand-new workforce of hundreds of thousands.

Every one bore the brunt of these increased costs. On September 10, 2001, there was no Department of Homeland Security, but was born soon after. Today, that department is a cabinet post with a multi-billion dollar budget. Adopting InfeXBloc™ will have similar implications.

The cost of care is:

- Expected to be more for InfeXBloc™ architecture than before, given the hardware enhancements, the rigorous processes, and protocols, and strenuous extra work and responsibility assumed.
- It is a worthwhile topic to discuss if CMS should partially support such upgrades across the Senior Care industry.

Chapter 6: Why is InfeXBloc™ Safer?

We start this section by stating a principle in the Safety & Resilience Engineering domain that "safety is not the absence of failure, but the presence of capacity to deal with its consequences without uncontrolled harm."

In our context, we can state that in a senior care community

"Safety is not the absence of infection, but the presence of capacity to deal with the unpredictable arrival of infection from outside without letting it cause uncontrolled harm to the residents, caregivers and the community"

The Prism of Controls and Safeguards

We acknowledge that the arrival of infections into a Senior Care community from outside is an unpredictable event. We do not agree with the idea (Heinrich's Accident Pyramid) that the frequency and severity of events is related. Thus, it follows that our traditional solutions for safety to prevent lower severity events are not enough to prevent uncontrolled harm from unpredictable high consequence events to our residents, caregivers, and communities.

In traditional safety thinking, there is a bias to prevention. The obvious statement goes something like this "every bad thing that happens, happens because we did not prevent it from happening". This statement is always true but is not relevant to unpredictable events. Prevention is attractive and important. It prevents a messy world from becoming messier. Prevention is so vital to our success that over time it has become a very large industry. We want to prevent everything bad from happening, so much so that over time we have become overly reliant on our prevention efforts. This overwhelming belief that prevention is the key to success has created a gap in our readiness for failure.

Prevention efforts cannot prevent causes that were unexpected just as planning cannot plan for an unexpected event. Prevention cannot prevent anomalies in our normally stable systems. Prevention, then, is not a control or a barrier for anomalous events. Prevention is not a safeguard against the consequence of a significant event. There is a significant bias that when something bad happened, it happened because we failed to prevent it. This bias is harmful to our business and prohibits us from being prepared to respond in a recovering way to minimize the uncontrolled harm to our business system. I doubt that in 2020 you will drive a car that only relies on crash prevention or fly a commercial airplane that relies on the prevention of aircraft control system failure. The role that seat belts and airbags play in a car or redundant hydraulic control systems play in a commercial airplane is not prevention, but a recovery in case of an accident or malfunction.

InfeXBloc™ goes beyond the failed-to-prevent mindset. It is an operational architecture that distinguishes between unpredictable and predictable events. The arrival of infection from outside the community is an unpredictable event, while the spread of infection inside the community is a predictable outcome (Figure 30 - 33).

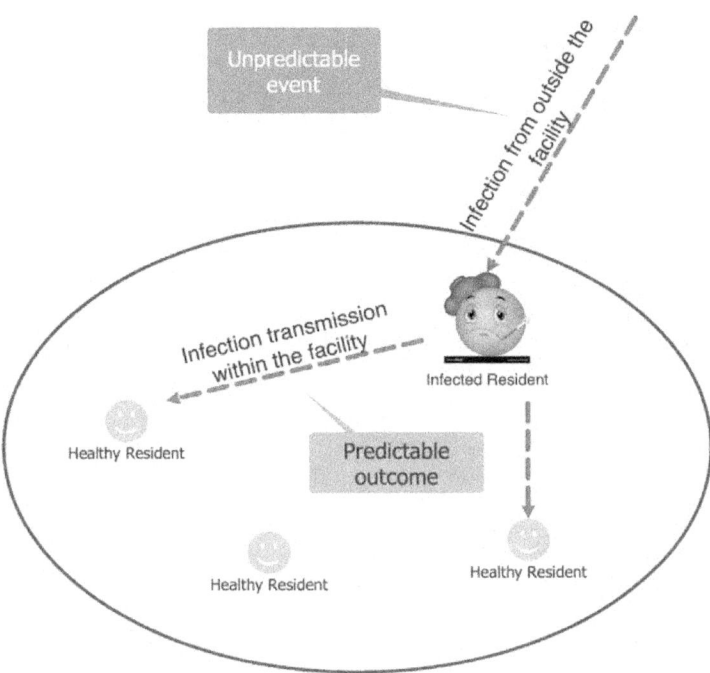

Figure 30: Without InfeXBloc^{TM}

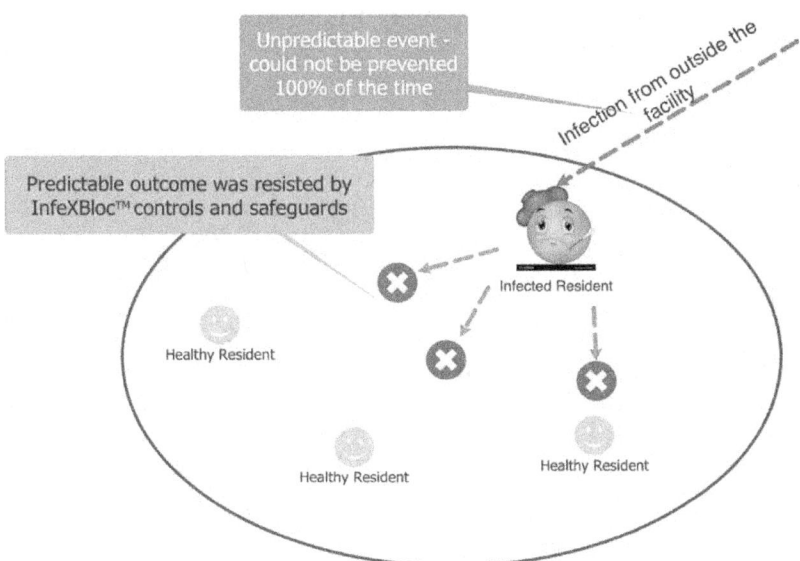

Figure 31: InfeXBloc^{TM} resists the spread

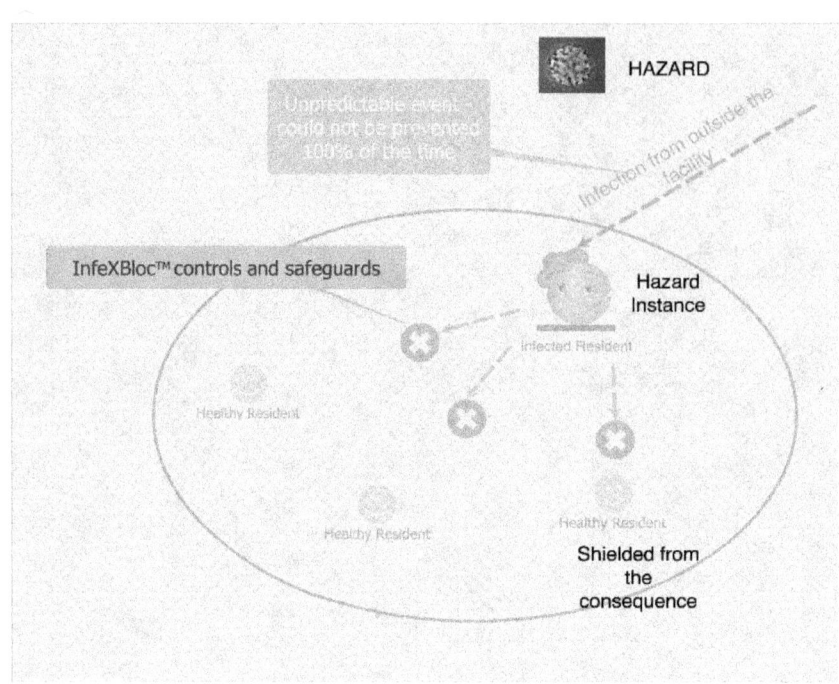

Figure 32: Explained in Safety Engineering terminology

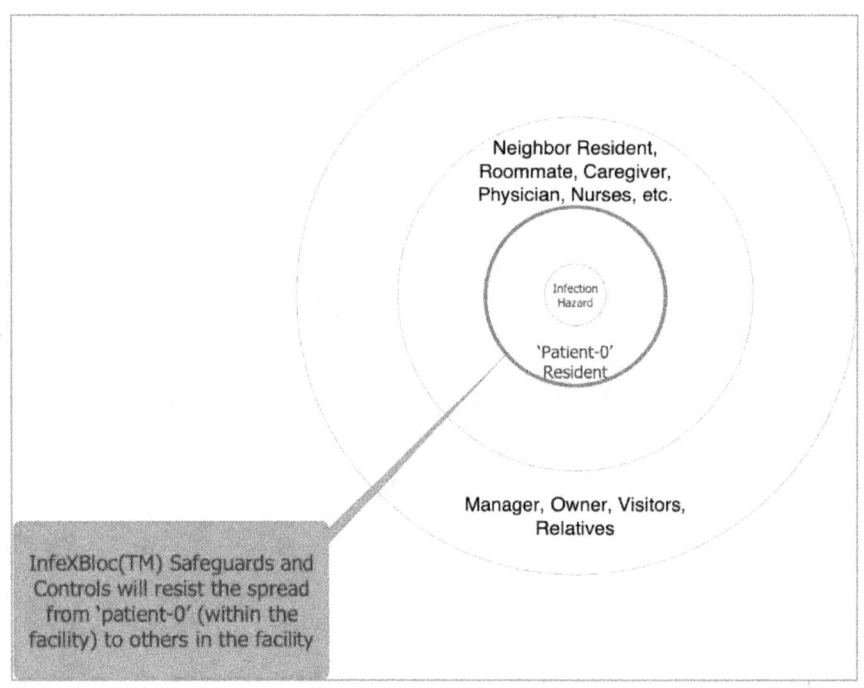

Figure 33: Primary, Secondary, Tertiary neighborhoods

InfeXBloc™ implements a combination of controls and safeguards to achieve the above results. In the section titled "Classifying controls and Safeguards in InfeXBloc™" we will categorize our recommendations.

InfeXBloc™ works at three levels

Overall InfeXBloc™ works at three levels:

- Planning for prevention
- Safe Execution
- Recovery, in case an infection enters the community

Planning for prevention

InfeXBloc™ recommends proper planning to prevent the entry of infection into a community.

- InfeXPASS™ system is an engineering control designed to prevent the entry of infection. When a relative/ visitor/ care professional/ supplier staff/ maintenance staff desires to visit the community, they use the electronic appointment system on the community website. That system asks basic health screening questions and records the answers.
- The above also applies to residents who may have been returning from relative visits, weekend outings, or Doctor's office visits/ hospital visits/ laboratory visits. This is intended to arrest the possibility of externally acquired infections from entering the community or if detected, appropriate controls are exercised.
- On arrival, a nurse validates essential health screening markers and issues an InfeXPASS™ that is valid for a specific duration. They are issued an access key which also controls the areas of the community that access is valid.
- The above access key also ensures that the visitor's current location within the community can be tracked in real-time.
- The above access key's ability to access community areas is tied to the InfeXCON™ condition of the property.
- InfeXCON™ is an isolation control designed to plan separation of hazards from people.

Safe Execution

InfeXBloc™ also recommends caregivers' proper PPE usage. There are controls to ensure that PPE is used as advised.

- Outside each resident room is a scanner that ensures that access is granted only if proper PPE have been used.
- By using InfeXCON™(an isolation control), we will allow for safer execution of care provision for seniors needing help with activities of daily living.
- Appropriate with the InfeXCON™ status of the community, these scanners can enforce door access and will also record events when the caregiver successfully achieves access.

- InfeXBloc™ also ensures that visitors/ supplier staff/ maintenance staff/ activity staff/ volunteers/ care professionals movements within the community as well as pertinent events are recorded.

Recovery, when infection enters the community

- When a resident acquires an infection from outside, and this is detected by one or more of these methods (Physician/ Care professional detection, Community Nurse, Caregivers, delayed lab reports, etc.), they are placed in quarantine in their room.
- Their room's negative HVAC system is engaged. All the rooms in the community are equipped with isolation characteristics. All trash in the room is disposed of in bio-hazard bins.
- Community InfeXCON™ status is turned to 'Brown' (this implies that this resident is quarantined and is not permitted to mix with other residents or staff). For other residents, community life stays as normal, meals are served in common dining areas, activities are happening.
- For the sake of the resident in quarantine, activities can be live-streamed to their room.
- The care giver responsible for the 'quarantined resident' is taking extra precautions suitable to the type of infection identified.
- When the resident's physician gives an all clear, resident quarantine is terminated and the community InfeXCON™ status returns to Green.
- Meanwhile, on a 24-hour cycle, all the resident's rooms and common areas are exposed to UVC light to achieve disinfection.
- All events of the InfeXCON™ status are streamed in real-time on the community website in an encrypted manner.
- If more than x% of residents are designated as 'quarantined' then the InfeXCON™ for the community switches to Yellow. What this means is that all residents are now encouraged to be in their rooms, the quarantined residents receive extra cautionary care, all room doors automatically stay closed.
- When any resident is declared COVID positive, the condition of the community is switched to Red, all trash in the room is treated bio-hazard, all rooms negative HVAC system is engaged, common room activities are suspended, meals are served in rooms. Caregivers and professionals exercise the highest level of precautions and PPE to ensure containment.
- Rooms in the community (in Golden Springs Ranch 24 rooms) will have the capability of containment for a COVID positive resident.
- All rooms are swept with UVC disinfection every 24 hours.

Quantitative analysis

Quantitatively, we can look at the number of transmission vectors activated in the daily care of just one resident. We assume that:

- *Each resident requires a care visit by a caregiver once every two hours. Thus daily, the caregiver visits the resident's room 12 times. For each visit, the caregiver opens and closes the room door twice (once during entry and next during exit). Thus, daily the number of touches that caregiver has with the doorknobs = 48*
- *Each resident leaves the room for breakfast, lunch, dinner, and one additional activity. So, the number of times the resident may interact with the doorknob will be = 16*
- *Each resident uses the restroom once every 3 hours. Thus daily the number of touches = 32. (If the caregiver is assisting in restroom/showering activities, then these interactions may be executed by the caregiver.)*
- *Each resident uses faucets 16 times daily, flushes toilets 8 times daily, and uses grab bars 8 times daily.*

Altogether, we can easily assume that the number of times that an infection transmission vector is invoked = 128 times.

Now imagine the community had 20 beds:

- The total number of active infection transmission vectors = 20*128 = 2,560

Now assume that one resident becomes 'infectious':

- The community will go to InfeXCON™ 'Yellow' and that resident's room will deploy the negative HVAC feature and all doors will be closed automatically. From that point, doors will open in a touch-free mode (nicknamed 'Star Trek' doors).
- Thus by designating InfeXCON™ 'Yellow' we have reduced the number of active infection vectors in the care of the other 19 residents.
- Assuming a 6:1 ratio of residents to caregivers
    - protecting the 'infectious' resident from the other 19 residents
        - will lower cross-transmission possibilities by 83.3% (640 infection vectors isolated from a total of 768 infection vectors)
    - protecting the 19 residents from the 'infectious' resident
        - will lower the cross-transmission possibilities by 16.6% (128 infection vectors isolated from a total of 768 vectors)
- Assuming a 12:1 ratio of residents to caregivers
    - protecting the 'infectious' resident from the other 19 residents
        - will lower cross-transmission possibilities by 91.6% (1,408 infection vectors isolated from a total of 1,536 infection vectors)
    - protecting the 19 residents from the 'infectious' resident
        - will lower the cross-transmission possibilities by 8.3% (128 infection vectors isolated from a total of 1,536 infection vectors)
- Assuming a 20:1 ratio of residents to caregivers
    - protecting the 'infectious' resident from the other 19 residents
        - will lower cross-transmission possibilities by 95% (2,432 infection vectors isolated from a total of 2,560 infection vectors)
    - protecting the 19 residents from the 'infectious' resident

- will lower the cross-transmission possibilities by 5% (128 infection vectors isolated from a total of 2,560 infection vectors)

It's also important to note that the extent of risk reduction is related to the caregiver to resident ratio. As this ratio changes, so does the risk reduction.

Table 1: Lowering of cross-transmission risk by deploying touch-free technologies

Caregiver to resident ratio	Lowered risk of cross-transmission for Infectious resident	Lowered risk of cross-transmission for healthy residents
6:1	83.3%	16.6%
12:1	91.6%	8.3%
20:1	95%	5%

By tabulating all of the results, we can come to some very important conclusions:

1. Deploying such technology significantly dampens the cross-transmission possibilities across the board.
2. However, the resident to caregiver ratio impacts the two populations differently:
    a. Deploying the technology lowers the risk for the infectious resident more when the caregiver to resident ratio is higher, but the healthier residents receive lesser protection. Hence <u>deployment of technology is more beneficial to the infectious resident</u>.
    b. Deploying the technology lowers the risk for healthier residents more when the caregiver to resident ratio is lower, but the infectious resident receives lesser protection. Hence <u>deployment of technology is more beneficial to healthier residents</u>.

In either case, deployment of multiple technologies reduces the extent of infection cross-transmission for all involved, making the community a safer environment.

Interestingly, when we go from one 'infectious' resident to two or more 'infectious' residents, the level of risk mitigation remains consistent, with no success reduction. This is because by adopting the 'proven trust' architecture, we have implemented 'micro-segmentation'. From an infection security perspective:

- In the current Senior Care community model, the blast radius of the infection is the entire community.
- In the InfeXBloc™ community, the blast-radius is confined to a single resident room. This allows the community to achieve maximum cross-transmission resistance at the first appearance of an infection. Therefore, any additional resident becoming 'infectious' does not raise the threat for the healthier ones beyond the initial level.

This fact means that the adoption of the InfeXBloc™ architecture helps us become "anti-fragile".

Comparative analysis

Examining the issue qualitatively, we can see another contrast form between existing Senior Care community and the InfeXBloc™ architecture, even when only looking at infection transmission resistance characteristics.

Category	Existing Senior Care community	Communities with InfeXBloc ™	Responsibility shared with
Paradigm	Everyone is safe unless they exhibit unsafe symptoms	Everyone is unsafe unless they prove they are safe via a repeatable process	
Paradigm	"Castle-and-moat" defense	Each resource (resident's room) defends itself	
Paradigm	The outer perimeter was the line of defense; the Entire community was defended at the outer perimeter	The perimeter has collapsed; micro-segmentation in effect; Outer perimeter as well as micro-perimeters are defended	
Paradigm	Either the entire community was 'safe' or the entire community was 'unsafe'	The community can sustain 'safe' even if some rooms are 'unsafe'	
Infection entry and cross-transmission resistance	The infection has an unchecked pathway into the community	The infection has no default entry into the community. Someone can still trick our entry checks, but that would be a deliberate act to deceive	Every entrant has signed off on their "InfeXPASS"
Infection entry	No responsibility assumed by the community if the infection enters the community	Shared responsibility of screening assumed by the community	Licensed professionals (Doctors / RNs/ LVNs) Business vendors (licensed & bonded)
Cross-transmission resistance	No responsibility of cross-transmission of infection assumed by the community	Shared responsibility for transmission-resistance assumed by the community. The best effort made by leading technologies.	Vendors of technologies
Cross-transmission resistance	If the resident is sick with an infectious disease, he/she could transmit it by default	If the resident is sick with an infectious disease, the infection can be contained. He/She could still violate community policies and cause transmission, but the threat is lowered	
Infection entry	If the caregiver is sick with an infectious disease, he/she could bring the infection in	If the caregiver is sick with an infectious disease, the entry checkpoint will present resistance	
Infection entry	The community does not do any work of screening non-residents	The community explicitly takes on work of screening at the entrance to grant/deny InfeXPASS ™	
Resists aerial spread	The community does not clean contaminated air	The community does clean contaminated air	

Category	Existing Senior Care community	Communities with InfeXBloc ™	Responsibility shared with
Surface contamination	The community does not clean surfaces with UV lights	The community does clean surfaces with UV lights	Patented UVC technology
Resists aerial spread	The community does not take responsibility for contaminated air circulating via the HVAC system	The community does take responsibility for preventing contaminated air from recirculating via the HVAC system	
Resists aerial spread	The community does not have negative pressure HVAC, hence infection can travel in corridors	The community does have negative pressure HVAC, hence infection cannot travel in corridors	
Resists accidental contamination	The community's resident rooms doors do not indicate if the occupant is 'infectious'	The community's resident room door indicates if the occupant is 'infectious'	
Least privilege principle	Community resident rooms do not have a default deny disposition	Community resident rooms can have a default deny disposition depending on InfeXCON™	
Enforcement	The community does not have to enforce PPE usage, only suggests it to caregivers	The community does enforce PPE usage	
Isolation	The community does not have isolation rooms	The community does have isolation rooms	
Transparency	The community does not have an InfeXCON™ status - hence no infection-related precaution escalation mechanism	The community does have an InfeXCON™ status and precautions will be escalated from Green --> Yellow --> Red	
Transparency	The community has no formal notification for staff, visiting family and guests, contract service providers, visiting professionals of any present 'infection'	Community explicitly notification for staff, visiting family and guests, contract service providers, visiting professionals of any present 'infection'	
Transparency	The community does not inform the family that some infection is present in the community	The community will notify the family that some infection is present in the community	
Transparency	The community does not have a Scorecard to convey its infection control posture	The community has an InfeXBloc Scorecard ™ - which allows for customers, regulators, and the community to gauge infection preparedness	
Resists cross-transmission	The community has doorknobs, faucets, flushes which are infection transmission vectors	The community employs hands-free faucets, flushes, and doorways	
Resists cross-transmission	The community has no separate handling of biohazard waste	The community has separate handling of biohazard waste	
Resists cross-transmission	Community does not require tele-health visits when infection present	Community does require tele-health visits when infection present - as a protocol	
Staff friendly	The community does not have load balancing for caregiver's workload if one of their residents (in their rotation) turns 'infectious'	The community has load balancing for caregiver's workload if one of their residents (in their rotation) turns 'infectious'	
Human Factors	No formal approaches to analyze human errors	HFACS approaches implemented to analyze failures and incorporate lessons learned	

Classifying the Safeguards and Controls of InfeXBloc™

Earlier in the section titled "Hierarchy of Controls" (Figure 14) we ranked the type of controls and safeguards in order of their effectiveness. We also noted that PPE is the lowest form of effectiveness against the Coronavirus and other infections. They are the last line of defense.

It is worth noting that as a community's process matures, it can add more controls belonging to each of these 5 hierarchy sections. The more safeguards and controls that are incorporated in the higher sections the higher the level of safety the community can offer. We expect this to be an continuous improvement list as newer processes, technologies and PPE become available.

We now will classify the controls and safeguards in the InfeXBloc™ architecture that are proposed to improve the effectiveness of safety.

Type of Control	Control or Safeguard
Elimination	No known way to eliminate the Coronavirus or any of the other infections that harm our senior residents
Substitution	No known way to substitute Coronavirus or any of the other infections that harm our senior residents with other less harmful bugs. Vaccines have some promise, but the efficacy of vaccines in our context is questionable at best. Vaccines are known to be less effective for the senior age group who may have many underlying comorbidities and conditions that compromise their immune systems. Many of the infections we experience in our communities have had vaccines available for decades and we still experience outbreaks.
Isolation Controls	Each room will be single occupancy and isolation capable
Engineering Controls	<ul><li>Negative HVAC rooms designed to prevent the escape of the bug outside of the resident's room</li><li>Touch free doors</li><li>Touch free faucets</li><li>Plexiglass visitation booths</li><li>UVC lights sweep every 24 hours cycle</li><li>Universal entrance complex</li><li>InfeXPASS™ entrance criteria</li><li>Thermal scanners</li><li>Access keycards for caregivers</li><li>PPE enforcement using scanners</li><li>Community has a real time InfeXCON designation</li><li>Encrypted event streams are published in real time</li><li>Video surveillance</li><li>RTLS (Real time location services)</li><li>Circadian Lighting</li><li>Pool fencing</li><li>Magnetic door locks</li><li>Smoke control sections</li><li>Fire exit doors</li><li>ADA compliance characteristics</li><li>All ADL events, caregiving events, medication delivery events are logged</li><li>Only community mobile phones are used on the premises</li><li>Self-service visitation appointments using Calendly™</li><li>Robotic tele-visitation with Physicians</li><li>In room group activities (e.g. Intercom-Bingo)</li><li>Enforcement of least privilege principle</li><li>Micro-segmentation of the community</li><li>Ability to correlate the three 'black boxes'</li></ul>
Administrative Controls	<ul><li>InfeXCON™ is an administrative safeguard mechanism</li><li>Safety dashboards are published in real time</li><li>Caregiver-buddy system to validate PPE usage</li><li>Sick leave provisions for caregivers</li><li>Group dining / In room dining option</li><li>Mandatory immunization program for caregivers</li></ul>
PPE	<ul><li>Masks</li><li>Face shields</li><li>Protective Gowns</li><li>Booties</li><li>Gloves</li><li>Alcohol disinfectants</li><li>Soap and water</li></ul>

One more orbit around the earth

In "Workplace Fatalities[35]", Todd Conklin quotes a fantastic example of how NASA created capacity in its process such that the ground controllers, astronauts, flight operations, etc. could have room to do problem solving in case an unexpected snag appeared during its space shuttle landing sequences. NASA designers did this by having the capability for the space shuttle to take one more orbit around the earth. This built in capacity in the process gave the workers additional time to problem solve rather than letting the unexpected failure create uncontrolled harm.

A long haul commercial jet flight is always loaded with enough extra fuel onboard to deal with unexpected events like weather or temporary airspace closure which allows the pilot to divert to an alternative airport in the neighborhood. By doing so, the airline creates extra capacity for the pilots, air traffic controllers, ground staff, etc. to deal with the unexpected event in a problem solving manner rather than allowing the event to create uncontrolled harm.

The above are examples of how systems that successfully do high consequence work in a stable manner always build in capacity in the process to allow its workers to have some room to do problem solving before and letting unexpected events lead to uncontrolled harm.

InfeXBloc™ is an operational architecture for a senior care community, that builds capacity in its process, to allow its workers the space to think in a creative problem solving manner rather than letting an unexpected event (like arrival of a deadly infection) to create uncontrolled harm. Sadly, senior care communities in Newyork, New Jersey, Pennsylvania, etc. had no such inbuilt capacity and the unexpected arrival of Coronavirus caused uncontrolled harm.

A learning organization

InfeXBloc™ community will implement the principles and approaches of Human Factors Analysis Classification System (HFACS) to distill lessons learned from what worked and what did not work from its daily operations in order to continuously improve its processes and systems.

The ability to correlate the digital 'black boxes' and produce a complete contextual picture of a failure event, allows the organization to learn about the patterns of events that lead up to a failure event comprehensively.

Chapter 7 : Delivering Transparency

Traditionally, senior care communities are not known for transparency. They have been more of closed-black-box-style operations where there is not much visibility into the operational internal details. The general format of operations is :

- relatives trust their elderly with the Senior Care community
- community takes care of them
- family members visit them whenever they can
- family members will be notified about Resident's progress

For all practical purposes, not much of what happens inside the closed-black-box is visible to the society outside. The government appointed LPA or Ombudsmen provide oversight but that is limited by the constrained resources and budgets of the Department of Social Services. Usually families make the decision of trusting their elderly in a Senior Care community's custody, with mixed emotions, relief and some guilt. Relief because their senior will be better taken care of, guilt because most of us would like to be able to take care of our elderly ourselves. Periodic visit to Mom's community is a good relief from the temporal guilt, our love and caring for our elderly. Usually daughters are thus more involved in the care of Mom at the community. When their elderly resident falls sick or refuses meals or has a fall or other unfortunate event, it creates significant stress for the relatives. The distance, inability to be with Mom, inability to see her or comfort her in her moments of distress creates a great amount of anxiety and stress for the relatives. Not having real time visibility or knowledge of Mom's progress greatly exacerbates the guilt and stress.

Interestingly, this closed-black-box nature of senior care communities really got further accentuated as the early response to the pandemic involved lockdowns, shelter-in-place, no visitations, etc. These necessary approaches while helping the public health authorities in 'flattening the curve' had their very adverse effects on the residents and their families. The pandemic and these remedial approaches have led to deaths of 55,000+ seniors, uncontrolled pain and suffering (Figure 34, 35) for the seniors as well as the relatives in their circle of care.

No one can undo the pain suffered or turn the clock back, but moving forward InfeXBloc™ will provide abilities for Senior Care communities to do their bit by opening up the closed-black-box. Apart from the infection spread control safeguards, InfeXBloc™ will also offer transparency as a significant way to lower the hardship for everyone involved in the future.

These transparency features will contribute to the benefits of adopting InfeXBloc™ as articulated in the chapter on "Benefits of Deploying InfeXBloc™ Architecture".

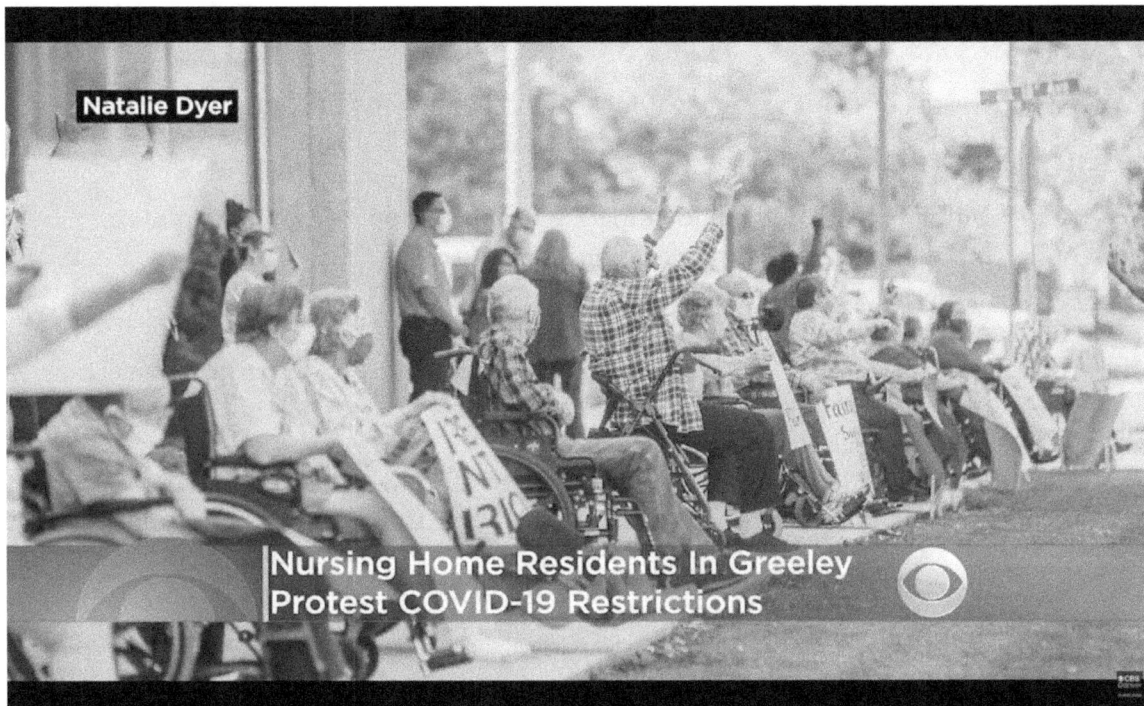

Figure 34: COVID-19 Restrictions have been very hard on seniors

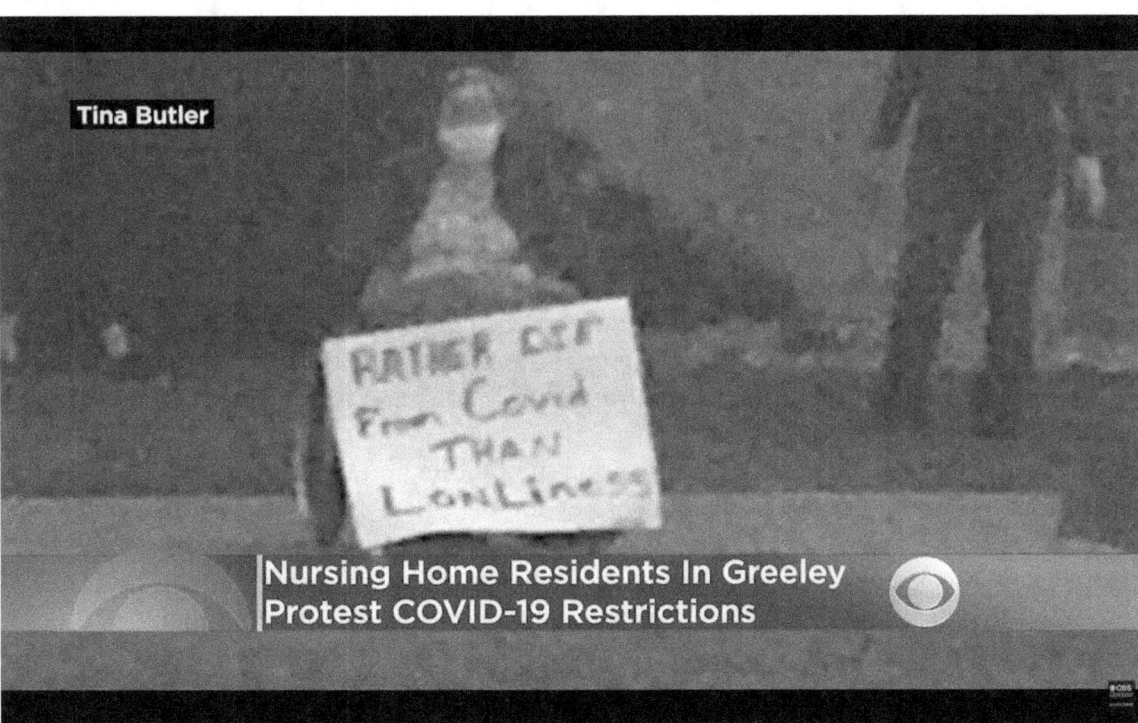

Figure 35: Death from COVID better than from loneliness!!

Mechanics of delivering transparency

InfeXBloc™'s mechanisms of delivery transparency will be via its mobile app. Without going into detailed technical specifications, here are some highlights:

- InfeXBloc™ Mobile App could be downloaded from the Apple/Google App Stores
- The Mobile App will require user registration
- Three levels of access are expected –
    - 'General User' is anyone from the public domain
    - 'Circle of Care User' is a user who has been authenticated as part of the care circle of a resident of an InfeXBloc™ community
    - 'Administration User'
- All access in the InfeXBloc™ Mobile App will be organized according to the above three levels with increasing access as we go from General → Circle of Care → Administration

Specific proposals to deliver transparency

While this will be a moving target, here are sixteen proposals that the InfeXBloc™ Mobile App will furnish towards the cause of transparency:

1. InfeXCON : This will be a real time Infection Control status of a community. For all users of the Mobile App, being able to see the current status of a community displayed on a geomap will be of great informational value. A first in the industry, it will allow various stakeholders to be informed and the value derived can be different. In all cases, we think it will be a positive.
2. InfeXPASS : This is the ability to obtain a entrance pass to the community. The availability of visiting pass application online will help streamline the process and make it convenient for visitors.
3. InfeXBloc™ event streams : The care events will be streamed in a encrypted fashion. The stream will be time lagged to maintain the operational freedom of the community. 'Circle-of-care' users could obtain temporary encryption keys to see details of their loved ones progress.
4. InfeXBloc™ - Care Bank : will be a screen on the mobile app that will allow 'Circle-of-care' users to review the details of each care event and possibly give a thumbs-up or thumbs-down review.
5. InfeXBloc™ Black boxes : Equivalent of black-boxes used in commercial airplanes, these provide the detailed chronology of event streams leading up to a moment in time. These provide privileged information to be used only by users with administrative access for forensic investigatory purposes.
6. InfeXBloc™ Stop Work Authority : is a special power vested to everyone at the community who operates at the sharp end. This authority allows the person to order a 'stop work' and insist an error be fixed. An example of this would be that when a caregiver sees her colleague missing a PPE step (washing hands / not wearing face mask, etc.), she is allowed to ask her colleague to 'stop work' and fix the misstep. The

InfeXBloc™ event stream will publish the instances of the invocation of this Stop Work Authority.
7. InfeXBloc™ - Chronic Unease : This is a principle that originated in the nuclear power industry and is a training offered to everyone at the community who operates at the sharp end and it encourages people to be constantly mindful of the hazards and risks in the community. The InfeXBloc™ event stream will publish every instance of the invocation of this training. With this, people will be aware of the mindfulness that the community teaches.
8. InfeXBloc™ Safety Dashboard – absence of negatives: This dashboard (Figure 38) will deliver a report (refreshed every night or more frequently) that presents metrics that are intended to deliver a message of absence of negatives events. In the world of Safety Science practitioners, this is generally referred to as SAFETY-1.
9. InfeXBloc™ Safety Dashboard – presence of positives: This dashboard (Figure 39) will deliver a report (refreshed every night or more frequently) that presents metrics that are intended to deliver a message of presence of positive events. In the world of Safety Science practitioners, this is generally referred to as SAFETY-2.
10. InfeXBloc™ - Caregiver Workload Spider : This dashboard (Figure 40) will deliver a view of the workload being experienced by a caregiver. When viewed over the shift hours it can help identify the pockets of time when the workload can be high or low. When comparing multiple caregiver's spider graphs, one can make reasonable conclusions about any asymmetry of workloads.
11. InfeXBloc™ - Resident Journey Map : This dashboard (Figure 41) will deliver a chronology of care events as a resident is being served at the community. These journey maps can be started at any point in time going backwards. One creative way of studying the state of a community by looking the journey maps of multiple residents side-by-side.
12. InfeXBloc™ - Resident 360 Map : This dashboard (Figure 42) will deliver a 360 view of care being delivered to her. The 360 arrangement can be based on types of ADL events being represented in the different segments of the 360 degree quadrants. Seeing this graphic it is feasible to understand the distinction between two residents whose care needs may be heavy in different quadrants (e.g. one resident needs higher attention with incontinence care, versus another with bathroom visits)
13. InfeXBloc™ - Dynamic PPE Inventories : This dashboard will deliver a listing of dynamic inventory status of PPEs at a community. This can be one indicator of the level of preparedness of a community.
14. InfeXBloc™ ScoreCard : This is a quantitative measurement system that will be refreshed every quarter and is designed to allow a viewer to get a relative measurement of how one community is faring as opposed to its peers. This is equivalent of JD Power ratings for automobiles. These scorecards will be audited by an independent third-party.
15. InfeXSIM™ - Digital Twin : This is a representative operational simulation https://youtu.be/lwVzNhLXLb0 of a community to allow seeing the effectiveness of InfeXBloc™ in curbing the infection spread risk. This can be used for marketing purposes to investors or prospective residents.
16. SCAN sponsored by InfeXBloc™ : This is a free monthly Meetup scheduled on first Sunday of each month at 6pm California time. The topics discussed here are related to the theme of 'Safety in Senior Care'. https://www.meetup.com/Senior-Care-Accountability-Network-SCAN

17. <u>InfeXBloc™ verified reviews</u> : Allow people at the sharp end (Caregivers, Nurses, Doctors, Administrators, etc. who are directly involved in caregiving) as well as the family and relatives to provide reviews of the community. These reviews will be verified and posted on the community's website.

Chapter 8: Can we prove this?

It is important to determine if the thesis presented in this book will work? Let us investigate.

Is the thesis theoretically sound?

- The notion of creating capacity in the process to deal with unexpected events is based on very sound thinking in the safety engineering domain.
- The notion of an exceedingly large attack surface area which grows astronomically with the number of beds is theoretically sound. Voluminous security research from NIST (National Institute of Standards and Technology) documents this for the cyber domain.
- The notion that we could never achieve 100% safety is also sound unless we live in a bubble.
- The notion that the 'castle and moat' paradigm will eventually always fail because we know infections can be airborne, infections can arrive from outside undetected and the nature of caregiving business involves direct human interactions and human error is a known reality.
- The notion that maximizing transmission friction is a way to slow down the transmission has been proven worldwide (by the strategy of social distancing, wearing masks, etc.)
- The notion that if there is a way to fight back, then an infection can be neutralized is proven in our own immune systems.

Has this thesis worked elsewhere?

The answer to that question is a resounding yes. This thesis has been proven to work in:
- the commercial aviation industry after September 11, 2001 terrorist attacks
- in cybersecurity for cloud-native software architectures
- the human immune system (a system that defends itself even when the enemy is inside)
- industrial safety systems that build incapacity in the process to prevent uncontrolled harm (e.g. seat belts and airbags don't prevent accidents, but prevent the event from resulting in uncontrolled harm)

Can we simulate this thesis?

Yes, we can. InfeXBloc™ is currently in the process of building such simulations (InfeXSIM™). These simulation models and their assumptions will soon be published.

None of this is overly ambitious because the simulation is a widely accepted methodology in epidemiological modeling as well as engineering fields as diverse as manufacturing, logistics, and space exploration. In fact, anywhere where live training or testing is too dangerous, expensive, or infeasible, simulation is the modeling paradigm employed (e.g. training a new jumbo jet pilot or landing the Mars ROVER). Over time, these simulations will be improved to offer enhanced assessment methodologies, for example:

- Given the type of friction mechanisms implemented, one could make reasonable assessments of the lowering of infection cross-transmission risk.
- The extent of impact these choices have on workforce productivity, PPE utilization, manpower costs, and overall operating costs.
- Over a period of time, it is entirely feasible to develop financial models for investors and insurance underwriters to correlate this degree of pandemic-resistance to the projected return-on-investment.
- Finally, it will be feasible to have management flight simulators, that can help owners, investors, and operators to plan a community with a projected pandemic-resistance level.

InfeXSIM™ - A new weapon system for the Senior Care Communities

InfeXSIM™ is a simulation technology that owes its origins to Prof. John Forester (MIT) who developed the science of systems dynamics beginning during WWII. In the modern era, this technology allows us to build, experiment and learn in a simulation environment, when doing so in a physical world is extremely expensive and/or risky. Industries like NASA, Department of Defense, Aerospace, Manufacturing, Supply Chains and Logistics, Oil and Gas, etc. use this technology extensively to examine and evaluate design ideas before they build.

For the Senior Care Communities, we see many use cases to deploy this technology. For example:
- We can examine the effectiveness of InfeXBloc™ to lower the risk posed by the infection spread vectors in a community
- We can build operational simulations to predict optimum resident to care giver ratios with various different optimization objectives (cost/ wait times/ load factors, etc)
- We can study the implications of seasons (summer -vs- winter) to predict the shift of infection spread threats on a community
- We can study the implications of a regional outbreak on the ecosystem of various Senior Care Communities
- If and when the next disease vector (COVID-xx) arrives, as soon as the scientists give us the features of the underlying bug (e.g. incubation period/ infection lifecycle/ transmission methods, etc.), we could simulate its effects on various Senior Care Communities
- We could simulate a Senior Care Community's supply chain to better forecast the need for PPE and not be caught flat-footed

It is safe to say that the InfeXSIM™ technology will present many opportunities for the Senior Care Ecosystem to be better prepared for the next bug.

Can we inject failure?

Failure injection is a well-practiced approach (from the science of Resilience Engineering) used in high risk high consequence domains. For example,

- often NASA astronauts practice with a deliberately injected malfunction (remember the movie Apollo 13, where astronaut (Kevin Bacon) responds to an injected failure during his simulation runs), or in the movie Crimson Tide where the Captain (Gene Hackman) injects a nuclear missile launch drill while the XO (Denzel Washington) is helping fight the fire in the galley.
- commercial jet simulators / DoD battlefield simulations deliberately inject failure to train the high-risk experts performing high consequence work
- Netflix uses failure injection using its Simian Army set of tools (Chaos Monkey, Chaos Gorilla, Chaos Kong, etc.) to simulate the failure of a data center/availability zone/AWS Region to test the resilience and fault tolerance of its systems.

InfeXBloc™ operational architecture will allow communities to drill by "injecting failure" to test the preparedness and resilience of the senior care community. This could be done by declaring that one or more residents have been found "infectious". Subsequently, all the actions taken by the staff, protocol switchovers by the community will be recorded. At the end of the drill, the 'black box' data traces will be studied to see the effectiveness of the protocols, practices, tools and training. The results of such drills are published on the community's website. It goes without saying that the resident who was declared "infectious" was only for the drill purposes and he/she and her relatives will know this secretly.

Can we establish the soundness by doing pilot projects?

In fact, that is the only way to prove the success of such a program. Just like NASA had to send many unmanned probes and 4 manned missions to the moon, before the successful human landing of Apollo 11, InfeXBloc™ will also go through 12-24 months of a pilot program.

During this time extensive data will be gathered, challenges will be encountered, tradeoffs will be considered and made, and decisions will be documented. InfeXBloc™ proposes to publish periodic blog updates of these pilot projects including final implementation reports. Further, InfeXBloc™ will continue to research this topic and upgrade the architecture and will make a knowledge base available for communities that deploy this architecture.

Chapter 9: Benefits of deploying the InfeXBloc™ architecture

Deploying the InfeXBloc™ architecture answers the question of how Senior Care communities can respond in order to protect their residents, regain the trust of families, the community, and the society as a whole, and continue to operate in a post-pandemic world.

Benefits of deploying the InfeXBloc™ architecture include:

For every stakeholder in this industry

- A concrete proposed strategy to tackle the big question about vulnerability to infection spread events like the pandemic. This is a strategy to build a 'Shield for Mom'.
- A set of proposals of transparency to invite the entire society to have an operational view inside a senior care center.
- A set of proposals that will allow regulators to be aware in real time the state of operations of a community.
- A new simulation technology approach to be better prepared for the future bug

For residents and families

- Residents and families will feel safer after the Coronavirus pandemic with InfeXBloc™ in place (refer to the previous section "Why is InfeXBloc™ safer?").
- Residents and families will have real-time visibility into the InfeXCON™ status of the community caring for their loved one and instantly be alerted to the fact that enhanced safety protocols have been initiated. After the community downgrades its InfeXCON™ status, the collective stress relief felt will be priceless.

For single community operators

- Single community operators can provide safer environments for residents (refer to the previous section "Why is InfeXBloc™ safer?").
- Single community operators will have higher personal satisfaction that they have done the best for their residents.
- Single community operators that are not InfeXBloc™ and have a resident who contracts an infectious disease are currently obliged to transfer the infected resident to a hospital. If there is an InfeXBloc™ community with an isolation room nearby, the community could consider transferring the resident to that community (based on a mutual contractual agreement). This has several advantages rather than relying on a hospital if all the resident needs is quarantine and do not require critical care:
    - Other residents are protected.
    - The 'infectious' resident is ensured to get the quarantine care he deserves.

- The infectious resident is protected from the additional exposure and higher risks involved in hospitalization.
- The Medicare/Medicaid cost of care at an InfeXBloc™ community can be lower than a hospital stay.
- Hospital overcrowding from non-threatening situations is prevented.
- At the end of the quarantine period, the resident can be transferred back to the original Senior Care community.

For multi-community operators

- Multi-community operators can provide safer environments for residents (refer to the previous section "Why is InfeXBloc™ safer?").
- Multi-community operators can make informed decisions about deploying shared resources across owned communities (e.g., Should their caregiver who works full-time in 'Community A' work overtime in 'Community B' if Community B is operating at InfeXCON™ level 'Yellow'/'Red'?).
- Multi-community operators have personal satisfaction that they have done the best for their residents to ensure their health and safety.

For DSS & Public health authorities

- When InfeXBloc™ architecture is adopted at scale, DSS gains the ability to know in real-time whether a significant number of communities in a geographical area are turning from 'Green' → 'Brown' → 'Yellow' → 'Red', indicating an infection trend. This real-time visibility can:
  - Allow DSS to share alerts across the geographical area.
  - Share expert recommendations to communities in that area.
  - Mobilize resources, as necessary.

This real-time dashboard will allow DSS to deal with a fast or silently spreading infection, without delay in order to thwart an impending crisis, in essence, functioning like an early warning system (e.g., Tsunami warning system).

- The hospital infrastructure will be better protected from any future surges of demand due to infection spread (see Figure 8 and 9).
- Governments will gain the satisfaction of having provided superior care for the hundreds of thousands of senior citizens under their care and oversight.

For Caregivers and Healthcare professionals

- A caregiver's career path is enriched when he/she has on-the-job education and experience in serving in InfeXBloc™ communities.

- Everyone in direct caregiving (Caregivers, Med-techs, Nurses, Doctors, etc.) will have a sense of fulfillment when able to meaningfully serve a resident(s) who may be experiencing infections with a lower risk of contracting the disease themselves. This can contribute to lowering and ultimately eliminating any stigma associated with the infection.

For Entrepreneurs, Community Owners, Operators, Investors, and business planners

The adoption of InfeXBloc™ architecture can be expected to deliver:

- a demonstrably safer community for senior residents and their families with a quantifiable proof point for the assertion
- a sound defense in the event of arising legal liability
- a certifiable audit that creates a strong viable evidentiary trail
- a simulation proof point to justify the investment
- a real-time visibility of the InfeXCON™
- a balanced scorecard (InfeXBloc Scorecard™) to achieve quarterly ratings to brag on
- a codified measurement mechanism to assess the value of a business
- transparency to the stakeholders (residents, relatives, staff, regulatory and overseeing authorities, society-at-large, etc.)
- get a forum to daily contribute with the pilot program updates. Being the first of its kind, we know that this will become a highly observed forum
- become contributors to the establishment of the InfeXBloc SCAN™ (Senior Care Accountability Network)

If we contrast the impact of InfeXBloc™ on the business model before and after InfeXBloc™ adoption (Figure 36), it is clear that the fundamental business model stays the same, but:

- a new and important value proposition for residents and their families is added.
- new information channels are added.
- new key activities, key resources, and cost structures are added.
- new revenue opportunities are included. The 'InfeXCON™ surcharge' could be an additional fee assessed for residents which will be related to the duration in a month that the community's InfeXCON™ status was elevated to Yellow or Red.

Overall the value delivered to all the customer segments is superior to the current model.

Key Partners	Key Activities	Value Propositions	Customer Relationships	Customer Segments
- Health care professionals (Doctors, Nurses, etc.) - Hospitals - Hospice agencies - Placement agencies - Hiring websites - Screening services - Suppliers	- Caregiving (ADL) - Activities (wellbeing, entertainment, etc.) - Adherance to compliance requirements - Home maintenance - Extra cleaning/ disinfecting	- Provide safe, happy, home living experience - Provide dignified living - Provide non-acute rehabilitative living - Take care of my mom and help me get my life back - Provide higher safety against infections - Improved resilience to the community's healthcare infrastructure	- Visitation - "state of Mom" reports - "INFCON" updates - "MedVisa" requirements	- Residents - Family of resident - Hospice company - Hospitals - Other RCFE - Community (senior healthcare ecosystem) - Oversight agencies
	Key Resources - Staff - Home - Capital - Oversight resources (LPA, Ombudsman, etc.) - Negative HVAC rooms - Isolation rooms		Channels - RCFE residence - Call center services - Isolation rooms - Digital diary of mom's care - Digital diary for RCFE	

Cost Structure	Revenue Streams
- Salaries - Debt service - Maitenance costs - Utilities - Capital to build Negative HVAC rooms, Isolation rooms - Extra salary costs for ehnahced caregiving effort	- Private pay monthly residence fees - Medicare/Insurance reimbursements - Monthly pay connected to facility 'INFCON' status

Figure 36: Comparing business model canvas[25] before and after InfeXBloc™ implementation

In Figure 36, black letters represent business model elements of the existing architecture - Senior Care community while blue letters represent new elements of the InfeXBloc™ architecture community.

** *Business Model Canvas is strategic management and lean startup template that was initially proposed by Alexander Osterwalder in 2008.*

For Insurance companies

- The InfeXBloc Scorecard™ will provide insurers with codified, quantifiable measures to define their underwriting criteria and objectively correlate insurance premiums. Such codification can then be extended to track the number of infections originating at the community. This can be used as an ongoing measure to assess performance.
- There is also an opportunity to linkup in real time with the 3 black boxes in the Senior Care Community to have visibility into events for forensic purposes in case of any claims are filed (such approaches are now available in automobile insurance industry).

Chapter 10: Challenges

With any real change in an industry's practices, there will be challenges in the implementation of InfeXBloc™.

- One of the big challenges is the acceptance of the notion that events like Coronavirus, are unpredictable. Unpredictable events cannot be planned for and prevented. But, we can prepare for their predictable consequences and prevent them from causing uncontrollable harm to our healthy residents, caregivers, staff, communities and business. This idea has very significant implications.
    - Community owners and entrepreneurs may resist the adoption because they would rather not have to deal with it. While this reluctance is understandable, in the face of possible or even likely long-term trust issues, it is worth reconsidering.
    - Building communities with extensive safeguards and controls to thwart the predictable spread vectors will require more capital investment.
    - Given the existing capacity in almost 29,000 communities which is 'pre-pandemic' in nature (meaning those communities cannot contain the uncontrolled harm), the task of retrofitting these communities is daunting, to say the least.
- Community owners and entrepreneurs may resist the adoption because they would rather not have to deal with it. While this reluctance is understandable, in the face of possible or even likely long-term trust issues, it is worth reconsidering.
- Residents and their families will also have to accept the improvements.
- Building communities with this infrastructure will require more capital investment.
- Human resources will require an initial as well as ongoing training. Caregivers will need to adapt to the improved protocols.
- When communities have more automated equipment, it automatically translates to more maintenance requirements.
- Regulators may need to consider the new paradigm – in California, it may even require a different designation than 6-bed Senior Care community.

However, it's also important to note that incentives could be a remedy for a number of the challenges discussed above.

Chapter 11: Implementation questions

Operators may have several implementation questions which we will try to answer here:

- Does InfeXBloc™ architecture have any pre-requisites in terms of the external ecosystem (e.g. electric cars needed a network of charging stations)?

    No. This architecture is entirely internal to the community.

- Can InfeXBloc™ architecture be implemented in increments or does it need a big bang implementation?

    It can be implemented in increments. However, the InfeXBloc Scorecard™ will reflect the partial implementation.

    Operators should think about this question using the framework in Figure 37. There are many variables that may have to be factored in to determine the approach e.g. ability to relocate existing residents, capital availability, cash flow, number of rooms, etc.

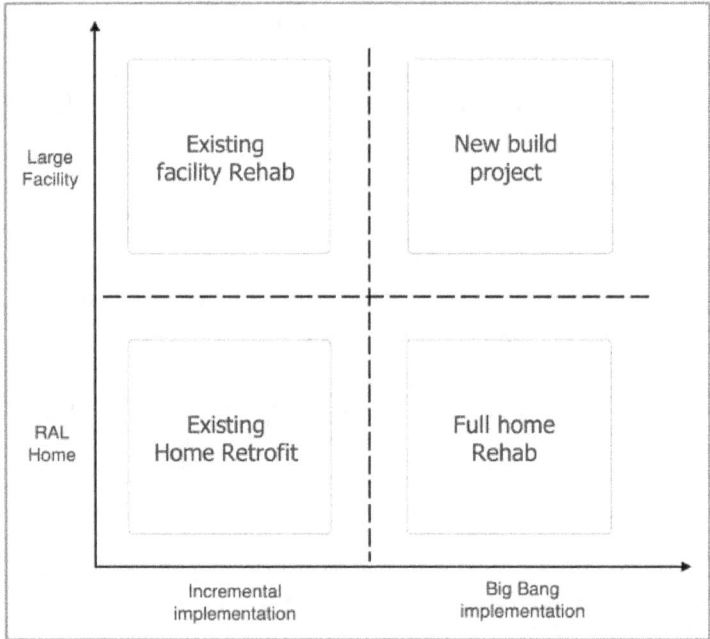

Figure 37: Implementation Framework

- Can InfeXBloc™ be implemented with some features using automation while other features being implemented manually?

    Yes.

- Are there parts of InfeXBloc™ that are so futuristic (e.g. Google Glass in 2011) that the market is not ready for it?

    No.

- Can an operator have some communities that implement the InfeXBloc™ while other communities are on older Senior Care community architecture?

    Yes. The operator should factor in various implications:

    - *On the brand image, customer perceptions, pricing variances, launch considerations (how, when, where, preparing the market for the launch, coinciding with competitor's launch dates, etc.)*
    - *How to prevent the Senior Care community part of your organization from competing with the InfeXBloc™ part of your organization?*
    - *A Beta release of InfeXBloc™ at a pilot community site*
    - *What are the implications on your back office organization (e.g. on call centers, purchasing, marketing) about a new product (InfeXBloc™ community) side-by-side of an older product (Senior Care communities)?*
    - *Observe the post-launch metrics via post-launch reviews (# of prospects, # of tours, # of move-ins, # of complaints, # of call center calls, etc.)*
    - *Watching social media feeds for prospect/customer/family feedback*
    - *If an existing community is being upgraded, define a migration plan from Senior Care community to InfeXBloc™ architecture community*
    - *Improvement release cycles (see section 'Implementing Change Management')*

Chapter 12: Digitization of Senior Care

Earlier, we agreed that safety cannot be measured. Unlike a physical object's capacity (our 5-gallon bucket), we cannot measure the Senior Care system's safety. We however, can measure other metrics and publish them in real-time in a transparent manner to foster the feeling of safety.

Using real-time dashboards

InfeXBloc™ enabled Senior Care community had a webpage that will display dashboards like Figure 38 – 42, that could help fostering the feeling of safety.

InfeXBloc™ Safety Dashboard
for Golden Springs Ranch, Palmdale, CA

Date : 08-21-2022   Current InfeXCON status : GREEN

	Today	This year
# of resident-days COVID-free	20	2,432
# of resident-days Infection-free	480	3,972
# of relative visits	7	537
# of medications safely delivered	79	39,564
# of tele-visits executed	12	729
# of resident-days 'fall-free'	326	3,972
# of room-hours of UVC light disinfection	38	597
# of InfeXPASS approvals / denials	21	645
# of hours of InfeXCON (G/B/Y/R)	24/0/0/0	536/0/0/0
# of 'patient zeros' that appeared	0	17
# of 'patient zeros' that caused spread	0	0

Figure 38: A real time Safety Dashboard – absence of negatives

Additionally, dashboards like the 'CareGiver Workload Spider' (Figure 40), 'Resident 360', 'Resident Journey' etc. will be illustrative of the actual happenings of the InfeXBloc™ enabled community.

InfeXBloc™ Safety Dashboard
for Golden Springs Ranch, Palmdale, CA

Date : 10-09-2022　　　　　　　　　Current InfeXCON status : GREEN

	Today	This year
# of successful ADL interventions	184	27,432
# of successful bathroom visit assistance	137	24,329
# of successful incontinence interventions	92	7,345
# of successful medication deliveries	57	3,972
# of successful meals delivered	45	4,537
# of successful Doctor tele-visits executed	13	9,564
# of successful Nurse visits executed	7	729
# of successful relative visits welcomed	9	3,972
# of successful vendor deliveries accepted	5	597

Figure 39: A real time Safety Dashboard – presence of positives

InfeXBloc(TM) Safety Dashboard
Golden Springs Ranch - Oct, 10 - 2020

Caregiver Workload Spider

Care giver : Sally Fisher

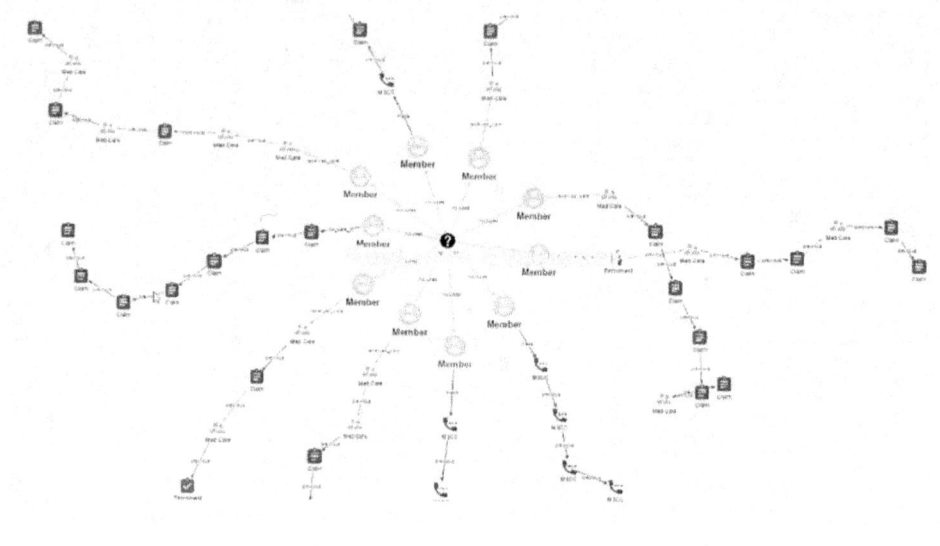

Figure 40: InfeXBloc™ Caregiver Workload Spider Dashboard

InfeXBloc(TM) Safety Dashboard
Golden Springs Ranch - Oct, 10 - 2020

Resident Journey Map

Resident : Doris Juarez

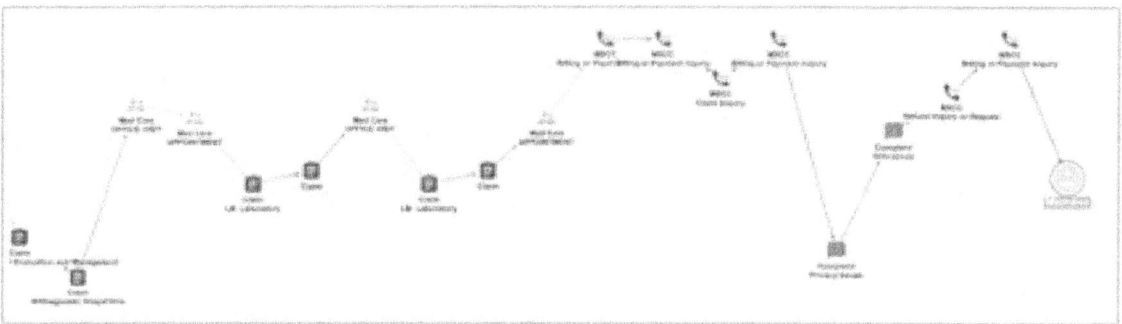

Figure 41: InfeXBloc™ Resident Journey Map

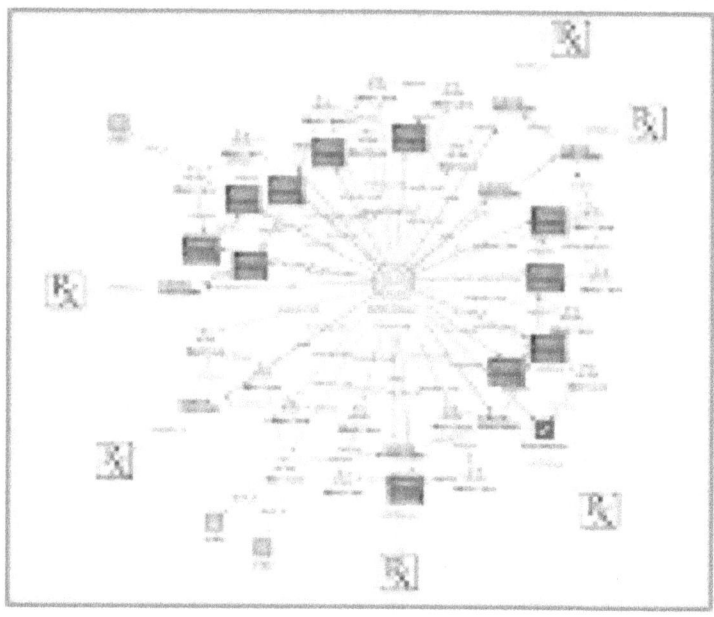

Figure 42: InfeXBloc^{TM} Resident 360 Map

Publishing a stream of events

We often emphasize the importance of documentation in a Senior Care community as a sustainable defense strategy against a liability lawsuit. Underneath that, is the desire to have an immutable chain of events that can paint a chronology to illustrate a diligent effort by the community. There is a variety of events that occur in a senior care community:

- ADL assistance events
- Medication delivery events
- Meal delivery events
- Activity events
- Hospital events
- Professional visit events
- Family visitation events
- Tour events
- Fall events
- To bed and wake up events

- Adverse health condition events
- Pictures were taken during events etc.
- Video streams published with time lag

If a Senior Care community could curate and publish, with time delay or in real-time, such a stream of events (Figure 43), it would go a long way to help relatives feel safe about their loved ones in our care. Needless, to say, we would need to take care of data anonymization to meet HIPAA compliance requirements.

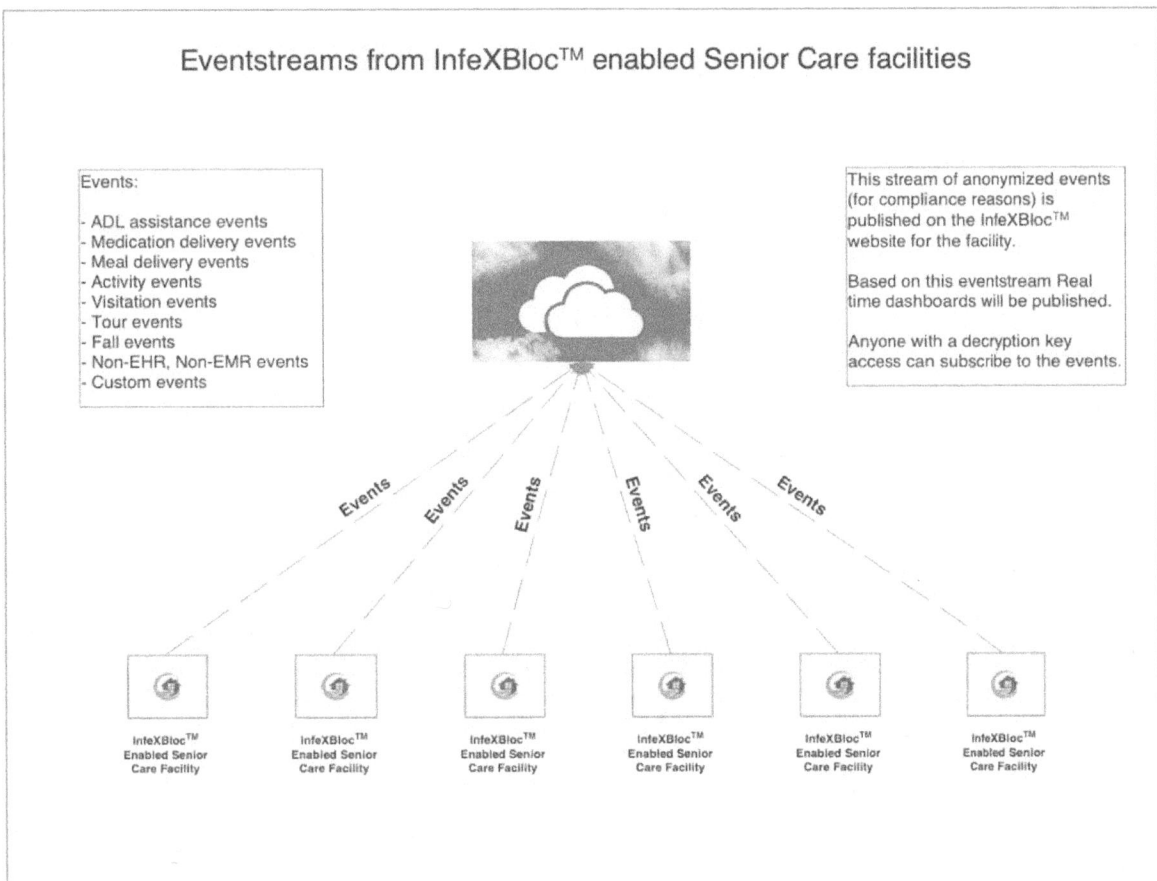

Figure 43: Event streams from InfeXBloc™ enabled communities

Implications for litigation

Every community owner or investor has a secret nightmare of the likely lawsuits that will arise out of this pandemic handling. If we read the tea leaves, Coronavirus litigation may make its Tobacco or Asbestos brethren look like child's play. While it is unclear how much help our Insurance companies provide or Congress provides with any umbrella protection, what is clear that regardless of the events of the last 5 months, we owe it to ourselves to build capacity for the future against this predictable risk. Publishing a stream of immutable events would go a long way. It would make our insurance companies very happy and they may even consider funding such efforts. They have already done so in the world of automotive insurance.

Implications for Licensing, Oversight, and Human Capital Management

Our LPAs and Ombudsman often have expectations that parallel those from attorneys. The oversight function is an important one to assure that our senior residents' rights are well protected. An immutable stream of events will go a long way to help this oversight function. More than anything, our caregivers could freely revisit their own event streams and assess their own performance. It would be relatively easy to report their own metrics.

Chapter 13: Future

Uphill climb ahead

In the aftermath of:

- 9-11, the aviation sector faced an unprecedented slump in airline travel demand.
- Publicly-exposed episodes of early internet fraud, the nascent e-commerce, and the banking card industry faced a daunting pullback because of mass fear about credit card/bank account theft, identity theft, etc.
- Publicly-exposed episodes of early cyber data breaches, the public cloud industry faced a massive pullback because enterprises were paranoid about the possibility of cyber-breaches and private data exfiltration.

The above, are examples of a massive trust deficit[3] among the customers – a trust deficit that always follows a catastrophe that was exacerbated due to a lack of preparedness (Hurricane Katrina is another prime example of how a catastrophe met with a lack of preparedness.).

Even if we assume that the Coronavirus itself was natural, the catastrophe that descended upon our seniors was a combination of that virulent bug and our poor infrastructure and deficient processes and procedures. The trust deficit[3] we are now facing (Figure 44) will translate to our uphill climb of convincing family members that our senior care communities are safe enough for Grandma or Grandpa. These difficulties may last far beyond the advent of a Coronavirus vaccine.

> Senior care programs are challenging during the best of times, but the coronavirus has made things worse. Nursing homes and other long-term care facilities have been a hotbed for infection from the virus, accounting for nearly 40% of deaths attributed to it.
>
> According to the Centers for Disease Control and Prevention (CDC), 8 out of 10 deaths reported in the U.S. have been in adults over the age of 65. These facts are making it hard for seniors to decide where they should go if they need long-term assistance, since the track record in nursing facilities for medical care is dismal.
>
> "People with loved ones in nursing homes, assisted living facilities, and other types of senior living facilities may be understandably concerned about their loved one's risk of illness from COVID-19," says the CDC, which offers guidance for older adults.
>
> Medical News Today reports that COVID-19 has hit older adults harder than any other age group. Underlying conditions and weakened immune systems make them more vulnerable to the ravages of the disease. Those suffering from dementia living in long-term care facilities present a specific challenge, since they may not understand the dangers of infection and forget to wash their hands or practice social distancing. According to the CDC, at least half of the older adults living in these facilities have Alzheimer's disease or some form of dementia.

Figure 44: Trust Deficit

We should examine the short term and long term implications of Coronavirus. In doing so, it's also worth assessing this topic based on the lessons we as a society learned from '9-11'.

- Short-term paranoia: In the immediate aftermath there is fear. We may see the impact on our market with a strong pullback in interest to let parents or grandparents choose to live in a Senior Care community. Many television interviews show relatives speaking to this effect.

- Long term apprehensions: The 45-60-year-olds of today (who are the key influencers of Senior Care resident's decisions) and their children (who will influence when the silver tsunami arrives in 6-8 years) will have the mental pictures of Coronavirus and its carnage in Senior Living communities fresh in their minds. Today news travels fast and bad news travels faster. All of these factors will have left long-lasting impressions on our customer's minds. These impressions will influence their decision making.

- Other implications: Experts on television tell us that, on September 11, a bunch of rag-tag jihadis plotting in caves in Afghanistan, launched a cheap operation (under $250,000) that not only killed 3,000 Americans but changed the aviation security landscape forever. That 'success' became a tonic for every malcontent with terrorism sympathies. The result has been an unstoppable 'war on terror' that has changed our lives, killed thousands more, and has cost us trillions. What is important to note is that military experts believe that terrorism is a cheap war to wage on America. These experts also say that bioterrorism is an even cheaper way to wage war. That prospect is a difficult one and the Coronavirus pandemic has brought it home.

The point is – do we have the architecture, infrastructure, processes, and procedures to resist the infection from spreading in our Senior Care community, regardless of the way it arrives?

Every industry is reinventing itself

Most of these causes of a trust deficit are either in the past or outside our control, however, regaining the trust of our customers is up to us. And, it can be within our reach if we take steps immediately.

Almost all industry business operating models have been touched by this pandemic. Every industry is scrambling to find solutions for the 'post-pandemic' economy:

- The tourist and cruise industry is working on new architectures.
- The restaurant and dining industry is implementing changes.
- The entertainment and casino industry is looking for ways to regain its momentum.
- The airline industry is looking for ways to reassure travelers.

The Senior Care industry cannot be left behind. We must reinvent. The "InfeXBloc™" architecture can help us do that.

Tomorrow will be better

On a brighter side,
- 9-11 did not fundamentally negate the rationale for the existence of the commercial aviation industry;
- bankcard fraud did not fundamentally negate the rationale for the e-commerce industry;
- cyber theft of sensitive data did not fundamentally negate the rationale for the public clouds.
- Coronavirus does not negate the rationale for the existence of the Senior Care industry.

Each of these industries served a need that transcended that industry's catastrophe. And each of these industries came back and continued to prosper after they were tested.

InfeXBloc™ can be used to work diligently with the help of the regulators and all participants in this complex ecosystem, to regain the trust of our customers by providing the best resistance against infection spread so that the Senior Care industry can continue to prosper as well.

InfeXBloc™ is a strategy that will employ several tactics and tools to achieve the overall goal of neutralizing the damaging effects of Coronavirus and other contagious diseases on our senior residents. As newer tactics and tools become available in this fight, this strategy will only become more effective. If a certain tool is deemed ineffective, it will be swapped out and a better one will take its place. The strategy will stay in force.

Applied Theory

Throughout this book, we have discussed the parallels between several different industries and drawn a common thread that runs through their operational architectures. We then extrapolated the architectural notion of "zero-trust" as a way to solve the challenges that were faced by those industries when their own catastrophe happened.

We now summarize this into a meta-framework that several industries can use to examine their domains and think of the operational architecture changes to approach this paradigm shift (from pre-pandemic to post-pandemic). We can sub-divide the universe of businesses into two groups.

group 1:   whose operations do not require that people congregate physically
group 2:   whose operations require that people congregate together

If your industry is in group 1, Coronavirus has had only a marginal impact on your operations. If your industry is in group 2, you have been impacted heavily by the lockdowns and the trust-deficit that will follow and your industry will require architectural re-engineering.

We have presented a solution that has been successful in both groups. Cyber-security in public clouds is an example of group 1 and Commercial aviation is an example of group 2. The notions of strong perimeter and zero-trust have been successfully used by both these groups. Above all, it involved a paradigm shift from an underlying security strategy of 'castle and moat' to a strategy of creating anti-fragility that assumes the enemy is already inside.

We believe that the Coronavirus pandemic is a landmark event and presents an enormous opportunity for disruptive innovation[11].

Industry Maturity Model

Most industries go through a maturation process which can last multiple decades. For example, e-commerce began in the '90s and has matured in nearly 24 years. What starts with low automation, negligible regulation, no standardization, a high instance of fraud, and overall low trust, eventually arrives at a place where processes are standardized, predictable service is achieved, and quantitative management and zero defect principles are practiced. Along the way, customers benefit from these improvements.

It's debatable where on this continuum (Figure 45), Senior Care as an industry lies. Nevertheless, the Coronavirus pandemic presents us with an opportunity to accelerate the maturity continuum in our industry. InfeXBloc™ architecture was designed to capture the momentum created by this pandemic to help move our industry up this continuum[23].

Once again, our customers – the residents we serve as well as their families and the communities we serve – will ultimately be the beneficiaries.

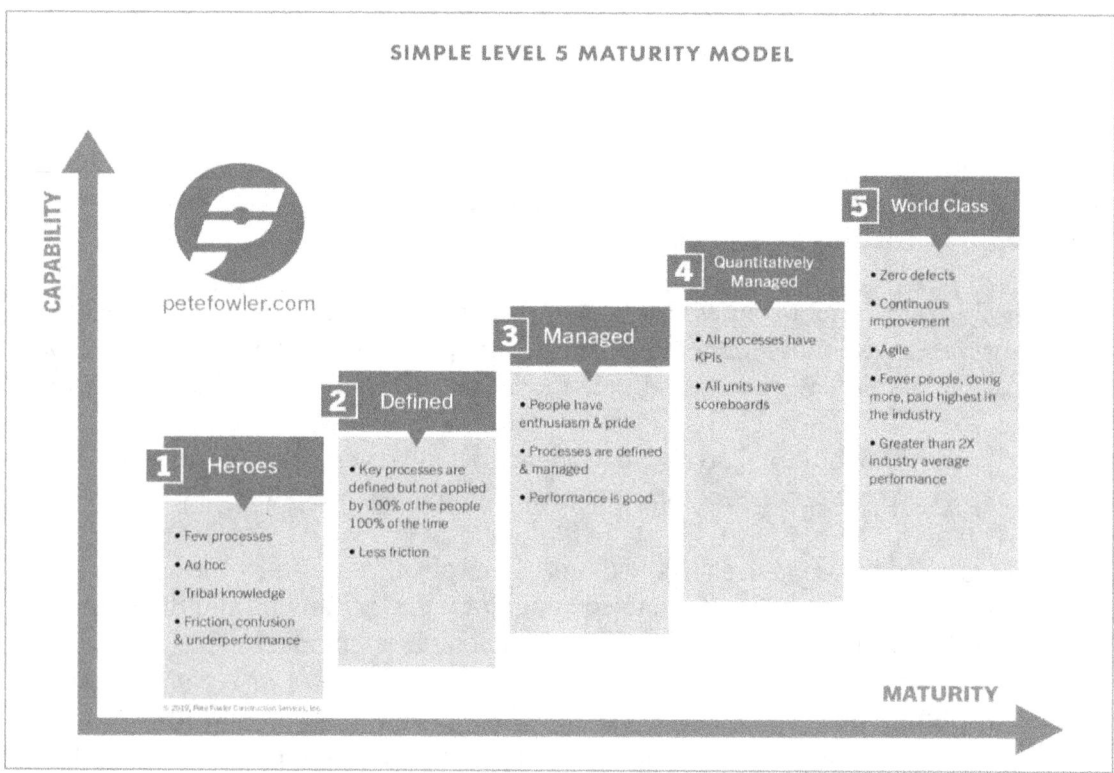

Figure 45: A 5 level Maturity Model

Chapter 14: A sincere hope

It will be a landmark day when not too far in the distant future, you are able to open a mobile app and see the real-time InfeXCON™ status of all Senior Care communities in a given geographical vicinity, all reported voluntarily!

On that day, we would be well on our way to regaining the trust:

- of our residents and their relatives
- of the communities we serve
- of the brave caregivers and healthcare professionals who help us in our service mission
- of the investors who trust us with their capital resources

A mobile app named InfeXBloc SCAN™ – Senior Care Accountability Network will help achieve this! This is the key to addressing a big concern voiced at a recent NIC webinar:

"Transparency is key," as Kurt Read, principal at RSF Partners, long-time NIC board member, and the current chair said, "whatever is going on right now will come out in the future, and those who are transparent and forthright in communicating what is going on will be viewed favorably once we get through the crisis that we're in now".

Chapter 15: The Care of the Caregiver

It is important to recognize the critical role played by thousands of caregivers in our Senior Care industry and the conditions they must operate in proximity to hazards like Coronavirus, Influenza, C-Diff, MRSA, Measles, etc. Despite 19 years of outstanding work, Julie Thao paid the ultimate price[39] when human error combined with multiple systems failure took the life of one of her patients. She teaches us an important lesson:

"Our hope is that Senior Care business leaders will recognize the critical responsibility to own and be accountable for the systems, the environment, and the culture the your frontline caregivers practice in. When the spirit of accountability and ownership does not exist among the leadership of an organization, then following a catastrophic event, the unprepared kneejerk reaction is one of fear, fear of litigation, fear of financial loss, fear of loss of reputation. This fear and unwillingness to take an accountable, systems-focused approach, forces the focus to the caregiver involved and to the unintentional error. It becomes necessary to blame them solely for what happened. If the individual is solely at fault and completely responsible, then punitive measures begin to make sense. On the other hand, in organizations where resident centric care, resident safety and doing the right thing are not just slogans and committee titles, but passions that live and thrive in the hearts of leaders, a very different predictable set of behaviors unfold, behaviors that courageously pick the pieces following a devastating incident, and stand together with the broken family, resident and caregiver, together, resisting the advice to limit transparency and disclosure and together begin the process of doing whatever is necessary to prevent this forever happening again in the future".

References

1. *A government watchdog report released on Wednesday found that eight in 10 nursing homes inspected were cited for infection-control problems and there were "persistent problems" when it came to infection prevention.* | *https://www.gao.gov/assets/710/707069.pdf*
2. *Protecting Nursing Home Residents from Infections like COVID-19. – WatchBlog: Official Blog of the U.S. Government Accountability Office https://blog.gao.gov/2020/05/21/protecting-nursing-home-residents-from-infections-like-covid-19/*
3. *Trust deficit https://www.newsmax.com/health/health-news/senior-care-long-term-community-pandemic/2020/05/26/id/969031/*
4. *Zero Trust - https://searchsecurity.techtarget.com/definition/zero-trust-model-zero-trust-network*
5. *OSHPD standard for isolation rooms https://up.codes/viewer/california/ca-mechanical-code-2016/chapter/4/ventilation-air#414.0*
6. *Simulation of Coronavirus infection traveling in the air across grocery store aisles https://www.youtube.com/watch?v=md6G2hqrhBE*
7. *Micro-droplet infection transmission. https://www.youtube.com/watch?v=H2azcn7MqOU*
8. *Blacklight simulation https://www.youtube.com/watch?v=MMwYsGews-8*
9. *Shortage of funds! (https://www.newsmax.com/headline/virus-outbreak-nursing-homes/2020/06/01/id/970004/)*
10. *For Seniors, COVID-19 Sets Off Pandemic of despair https://link.theepochtimes.com/mkt_app/for-seniors-covid-19-sets-off-pandemic-of-despair_3371290.html*
11. *Disruptive Innovation https://www.youtube.com/watch?v=qDrMAzCHFUU*
12. *Perspectives on the Pandemic: https://www.youtube.com/watch?v=UIDsKdeFOmQ&list=PLlGSlkijht5jFHF2o8rIhiOPHNT1OzyWE*
13. *The long regulatory road!! https://www.forbes.com/sites/howardgleckman/2020/06/09/how-to-redesign-long-term-care-for-older-adults-after-covid-19/#2dd0f21a5d85*
14. *Beyond Corp – by Google https://www.beyondcorp.com/*
15. *Riskiest Places to catch Coronavirus. https://www.foxnews.com/health/coronavirus-riskiest-places-contracting*
16. *Antifragile- by Naseem Taleb   https://www.amazon.com/Antifragile-Things-Disorder-ANTIFRAGILE-Bookback/dp/B00QORW08I/ref=sr_1_4?dchild=1&keywords=antifragile&qid=1592399231&sr=8-4*
17. *McKinsey report https://www.mckinsey.com/business-functions/organization/our-insights/reimagining-the-office-and-work-life-after-covid-19*
18. *We are fully compliant: https://www.buzzfeednews.com/article/rosalindadams/nobody-knows-exactly-how-hard-the-coronavirus-is-hitting*
19. *Causal Loop diagram for the threat of COVID-19 : https://www.thelancet.com/pdfs/journals/eclinm/PIIS2589-5370(20)30069-9.pdf*

20. Coronavirus cases in Senior Care Communities
https://www.cdss.ca.gov/Portals/9/Additional-Resources/Research-and-Data/DSSDS/6-19.pdf
21. CDC infection control recommendations
https://www.cdc.gov/infectioncontrol/basics/standard-precautions.html
https://www.cdc.gov/infectioncontrol/basics/transmission-based-precautions.html
https://www.cdc.gov/infectioncontrol/guidelines/isolation/index.html
22. Ground zero of Coronavirus
https://www.forbes.com/sites/theapothecary/2020/05/26/nursing-homes-assisted-living-communities-0-6-of-the-u-s-population-43-of-u-s-covid-19-deaths/#9cd470374cdb
23. Industry Maturity Model https://www.petefowler.com/blog/2019/5/1/maturity-model
24. Contagious diseases in USA https://www.ncbi.nlm.nih.gov/pmc/articles/PMC4175560/
25. Business Model Canvas https://www.youtube.com/watch?v=QoAOzMTLP5s
26. Coronavirus is airborne ! https://www.newsmax.com/us/who-coronavirus-airborne-spread/2020/07/07/id/976094/
27. Effectiveness of vaccines https://theconversation.com/how-effective-does-a-covid-19-coronavirus-vaccine-need-to-be-to-stop-the-pandemic-a-new-study-has-answers-142468
28. Competing against non-consumption https://www.christenseninstitute.org/blog/non-consumption-is-your-fiercest-competition-and-its-winning/
29. Effectiveness of Contact Tracing https://theconversation.com/contact-tracings-long-turbulent-history-holds-lessons-for-covid-19-142511
30. Will COVID-19 vaccine save the world
https://www.mckinsey.com/~/media/McKinsey/Industries/Pharmaceuticals%20and%20Medical%20Products/Our%20Insights/On%20pins%20and%20needles%20Will%20COVID%2019%20vaccines%20save%20the%20world/On-pins-and-needles-Will-COVID-19-vaccines-save-the-world-v4.pdf
31. Sabo techniques of Japan https://www.youtube.com/watch?v=HIkz-RC_Gho
32. Industrial accident in Bhilai https://www.groundxero.in/wp-content/uploads/2019/04/compiled-BSP-report-pdf_pagenumber.pdf
33. Safety as a presence of capacity – Todd Conklin
https://www.youtube.com/watch?v=_qo8hh_Rb1k
34. Hazard Identification https://www.osha.gov/shpguidelines/hazard-Identification.html
35. Workplace Fatalities https://www.amazon.com/Workplace-Fatalities-Discussion-Fatality-Reduction/dp/B07QV9YLJL/ref=sr_1_1?dchild=1&keywords=workplace+fatalities&qid=1599049274&sr=8-1
36. The Black Swan https://www.amazon.com/Black-Swan-text-First-Taleb/dp/B003TEOG9U/ref=sr_1_10?crid=UGDQ11O7LNU&dchild=1&keywords=the+black+swan+nassim+taleb&qid=1599165368&sprefix=the+black+swan%2Caps%2C213&sr=8-10
37. OSHA Guidance for preparing workplaces for COVID-19
https://www.osha.gov/Publications/OSHA3990.pdf
38. Human Factors Analysis Classification System
https://www.youtube.com/watch?v=LakltxjqbFc
39. The story of Julie Thao https://www.youtube.com/watch?v=0j-MScJM0So

40. *James Reason's Swiss Cheese Model of Accident Causation*
    https://www.youtube.com/watch?v=MfWpMrEOlJ8
41. *When the worst accident happens – Todd Conklin. https://www.amazon.com/When-Worst-Accident-Happens-catastrophic-ebook/dp/B089221K5X*
42. *Gartner's Post Pandemic Planning Framework*
    https://emtemp.gcom.cloud/ngw/globalassets/en/insights/postpandemic-planning-framework/gartner-postpandemic-planning-framework.pdf
43. *Strategies for Safer Senior Living Communities (American Institute of Architects) - http://content.aia.org/sites/default/files/2020-07/Building_Type_Report_Senior_Living_Final7_2.pdf*
44.

Bibliography

"3D Model Shows How an Indoor Cough Can Spread a 'Cloud' of Coronavirus." *YouTube*, The Telegraph, 9 Apr. 2020, 3D model shows how an indoor cough can spread a 'cloud' of coronavirus.

Adams, Rosalind. "Nobody Knows Exactly How Hard The Coronavirus Is Hitting America's Senior Care Communities." *BuzzFeed News*, BuzzFeed News, 18 June 2020, www.buzzfeednews.com/article/rosalindadams/nobody-knows-exactly-how-hard-the-coronavirus-is-hitting.

Allison, Lynn. "How the Coronavirus Affects Senior Care." *Newsmax*, Newsmax Media, Inc. Newsmax Media, Inc., 26 May 2020, www.newsmax.com/health/health-news/senior-care-long-term-community-pandemic/2020/05/26/id/969031/.

Alonso-Zaldivar, Ricardo, and Candice Choi. "Nearly 26,000 Nursing Home COVID-19 Deaths Reported." *Newsmax*, Newsmax Media, Inc. Newsmax Media, Inc., 1 June 2020, www.newsmax.com/headline/virus-outbreak-nursing-homes/2020/06/01/id/970004/.

"Black Light Simulation Shows How Quickly COVID-19 Spreads in Restaurants | NowThis." *YouTube*, Now This, 20 May 2020, www.youtube.com/watch?v=MMwYsGews-8.

Boland, Brodie, et al. "Reimagining the Office and Work Life after COVID-19." *McKinsey & Company*, McKinsey & Company, 8 June 2020, www.mckinsey.com/business-functions/organization/our-insights/reimagining-the-office-and-work-life-after-covid-19.

Bradley, Declan Terence, et al. "A Systems Approach to Preventing and Responding to COVID-19." *The Lancet*, EClinicalMedicine, 28 Mar. 2020, www.thelancet.com/pdfs/journals/eclinm/PIIS2589-5370(20)30069-9.pdf.

"Coronavirus Disease (COVID-19) Information." *Department of Social Services*, California Department of Social Services, 19 June 2020, www.cdss.ca.gov/#covid19.

"Coronavirus: New Facts about Infection Mechanisms - NHK Documentary." *YouTube*, NHK WORLD-JAPAN, 3 Apr. 2020, www.youtube.com/watch?v=H2azcn7MqOU.

"Disruptive Innovation Explained." *YouTube*, Harvard Business Review, 30 Mar. 2012, www.youtube.com/watch?v=qDrMAzCHFUU.

Gleckman, Howard. "How To Redesign Long-Term Care For Older Adults After Covid-19." *Forbes*, Forbes Magazine, 10 June 2020, www.forbes.com/sites/howardgleckman/2020/06/09/how-to-redesign-long-term-care-for-older-adults-after-covid-19/#2dd0f21a5d85.

Graham, Judith. "COVID-19: Seniors Struggle with the Psychic Pain of Despair amid Extended Restrictions." *The Epoch Times*, The Epoch Times, 17 June 2020, www.link.theepochtimes.com/mkt_app/for-seniors-covid-19-sets-off-pandemic-of-despair_3371290.html.

"Infection Control Deficiencies Were Widespread and Persistent in Nursing Homes Prior to COVID-19 Pandemic." *U.S. Government Accountability Office*, U.S. Government Accountability Office, 20 May 2020, U.S. Government Accountability Office.

"Isolation Precautions." *Centers for Disease Control and Prevention*, Centers for Disease Control and Prevention, 22 July 2019, www.cdc.gov/infectioncontrol/guidelines/isolation/index.html.

Miles, Frank. "These Places Pose the Greatest Risks for Contracting Coronavirus." *Fox News*, FOX News Network, 15 June 2020, www.foxnews.com/health/coronavirus-riskiest-places-contracting.

"Perspectives on the Pandemic | The (Undercover) Epicenter Nurse | Episode Nine." *YouTube*, Journeyman Pictures, 9 June 2020, www.youtube.com/watch?v=UIDsKdeFOmQ&list=PLlGSlkijht5jFHF2o8rIhiOPHNT1OzyWE.

"Protecting Nursing Home Residents from Infections like COVID-19." *WatchBlog: Official Blog of the U.S. Government Accountability Office*, 21 May 2020, www.blog.gao.gov/2020/05/21/protecting-nursing-home-residents-from-infections-like-covid-19/.

Rouse, Margaret. "What Is Zero-Trust Model (Zero Trust Network)? - Definition from WhatIs.com." *SearchSecurity*, TechTarget, 9 Apr. 2019, www.searchsecurity.techtarget.com/definition/zero-trust-model-zero-trust-network.

"Run Zero Trust Security Like Google." *BeyondCorp*, BeyondCorp, www.beyondcorp.com/.

"Searchable Platform for Building Codes." *UpCodes*, 2016, www.up.codes/viewer/california/ca-mechanical-code-2016/chapter/4/ventilation-air#414.0.

"Standard Precautions for All Patient Care." *Centers for Disease Control and Prevention*, Centers for Disease Control and Prevention, 26 Jan. 2016, www.cdc.gov/infectioncontrol/basics/standard-precautions.html.

Taleb, Nassim Nicholas. *Antifragile: Things That Gain from Disorder*. Random House, 2016.

"Transmission-Based Precautions." *Centers for Disease Control and Prevention*, Centers for Disease Control and Prevention, 7 Jan. 2016, www.cdc.gov/infectioncontrol/basics/transmission-based-precautions.html.

Roy, Avik. "The Most Important Coronavirus Statistic: 42% Of U.S. Deaths Are From 0.6% Of The Population." *Forbes*, Forbes Magazine, 29 May 2020, www.forbes.com/sites/theapothecary/2020/05/26/nursing-homes-assisted-living-communities-0-6-of-the-u-s-population-43-of-u-s-covid-19-deaths/#9cd470374cdb.

Fowler, Pete. "Maturity Models." *PFCS*, PFCS, 14 May 2019, www.petefowler.com/blog/2019/5/1/maturity-model.

Bruce Y. Lee Professor of Health Policy and Management. "How Effective Does a COVID-19 Coronavirus Vaccine Need to Be to Stop the Pandemic? A New Study Has Answers." *The Conversation*, 23 July 2020, theconversation.com/how-effective-does-a-covid-19-coronavirus-vaccine-need-to-be-to-stop-the-pandemic-a-new-study-has-answers-142468.

Ojomo, By: Efosa, et al. "Nonconsumption Is Your Fiercest Competition-and It's Winning." *Christensen Institute*, 15 Apr. 2019, www.christenseninstitute.org/blog/non-consumption-is-your-fiercest-competition-and-its-winning/.

Amy Lauren Fairchild Dean and Professor, et al. "Contact Tracing's Long, Turbulent History Holds Lessons for COVID-19." *The Conversation*, 16 July 2020, theconversation.com/contact-tracings-long-turbulent-history-holds-lessons-for-covid-19-142511

About

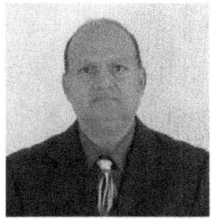

Ashish Warudkar is trained at

IIT Bombay	*Mechanical Engineering*
UCI	*Predictive Analytics (7/8)*
Harvard	*Disruptive Innovation Strategy with Clayton Christensen*
MIT	*Advanced Certificate for Executives in Management, Innovation & Technology*
	Architecture & Systems Engineering of Complex Systems
	Platform Strategy – Building & Thriving a vibrant ecosystem
	Business Dynamics – Diagnosing and solving complex business problems
	Executive Certificate in Strategy and Innovation
Product School	*Product Management*
BWW	*Network Marketing*
Oren Klaff	*Pitch Mastery*

He has worked in the software industry for 30+ years including 19+ years in the healthcare sector. He also has been an entrepreneur for over two decades and provides consultation to "Golden Springs Ranch" which is an upcoming InfeXBloc™ community in Palmdale, California which will introduce the innovations discussed in this book to provide its precious residents with a safe happy community and their families with peace of mind.

web	: www.InfeXBloc.com
email	: ashish@InfeXBloc.com , or ashish.warudkar@sloan.mit.edu
twitter	: *@InfeXBloc*
facebook	: *InfeXBloc*
Instagram	: *InfeXBloc*

©This book is a copyrighted work of Ashish Warudkar. All Rights are Reserved.
"InfeXBloc™", "InfeXPASS™", "INFEXCON™", "InfeXBloc Scorecard™", InfeXSIM^{TM} are registered trademarks of Pratibha Creative Resources LLC.

www.ingramcontent.com/pod-product-compliance
Lightning Source LLC
Chambersburg PA
CBHW081437220526
45466CB00008B/2425